MEDICAL SCHOOL: THE INTERVIEW AND THE APPLICANT

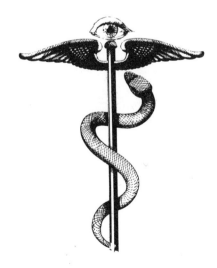

MEDICAL SCHOOL: THE INTERVIEW AND THE APPLICANT

MARGUERITE RUSH LERNER, M.D.

Professor of Clinical Dermatology
Yale University School of Medicine

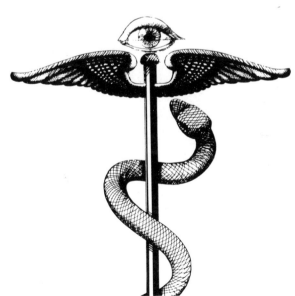

Barron's Educational Series, Inc./Woodbury, New York

All inquiries should be addressed to:
Barron's Educational Series, Inc.
113 Crossways Park Drive
Woodbury, New York 11797

Library of Congress Catalog Card No. 76-44368

International Standard Book No. 0-8120-0752-2

Library of Congress Cataloging in Publication Data
Lerner, Marguerite Rush.
  MEDICAL SCHOOL: The Interview and the Applicant
  Bibliography: p.
  1. Medical   colleges—United   States—Admission. 2. Medical
colleges—United States. I. Title. [DNLM: 1. Schools, Medical—United
States. 2. Students, Premedical. 3. Educational measurement. W19 L616p]
R838.4.L47   610'.7'1173   76-44368
ISBN 0-8120-0752-2

Acknowledgements

I want to thank Mrs. Waltraut F. Dubé, Associate Director, Division of Student Studies, of the Association of American Medical Colleges, for allowing me to use the data she compiled on medical school admissions.

Contents

Introduction

What *would you look for in a potential candidate for medical school if you were a member of the admissions committee?* An applicant-supplicant — and the applicants *are* supplicants unless their scores on the Medical College Admission Test are in the 80th to 90th percentile and their cumulative grade averages 3.7 or above — who assures you of his or her devotion to caring for the sick? One whose compassion for humanity knows no bounds, the eager doctor-to-be who has served as a candy striper or done yeoman's duty as a volunteer on the wards or in the emergency room? Perhaps the individual who declares a desire to work in Appalachia, to bring good medical care to the regions with a low physician-to-patient density? Or a seeker of just and equal care for the deprived of the cities?

And what about the searcher of the unknown who wants to expand the frontiers of medicine, who recognizes the requirement for infinite time and patience to focus on the small point that might lead to the discovery of the molecular basis of an illness or a congenital anomaly and who must have a background of medical knowledge and an association with patients in order to sharpen insights and seize inspiration?

People on the admissions committee at a medical school con themselves into believing that they are not being conned by the person who declares, ''I want to go to this medical school more than any other one'' or the cherubic man-child or woman-child who could move mountains if given the chance to become a doctor. Well-intentioned? Of course. Capable? Maybe. And the intended medical scientist might have neither the talent nor the persistence to pursue the unknown.

It is not unusual for an individual who has a record of offenses against society to stand before a court of law and say that he or she likes people and wants to help them. Although the number of persons with serious emotional problems applying to medical school is small, admissions people are wary about accepting applicants with severe personality disorders. The committee can fall back on the cliché, "All of us make mistakes." But they don't want to make mistakes. They want to select the best possible candidates for their school.

It is not easy to identify with precision on the basis of an interview what candidate is going to be an innovator or an achiever. Indeed, it is likely that the very lack of precision is responsible for accepting applicants who go on to great things. It is also likely that the same lack of precision on the part of the interviewers is what helps make possible a distribution of superior candidates to all medical schools instead of a few schools capturing all the wizards.

One would be a fool not to recognize the role of the admissions committee, and particularly its chairperson, in charting the course of the medical school itself. Perhaps second in importance only to the promotion committee, the group involved with admitting students is responsible for the selection of those who will practice the art and science of medicine and hence is indirectly responsible for the direction of advancement in medical science and care. It is not likely that any member of a medical school's admissions committee congratulates himself or herself for having made the right decision in each case because there is no one right decision. There are far more good candidates than places available. Many first-year classes of medical students could be duplicated with no loss in quality. The credentials of applicants to medical school are high.

In the chapters on the admissions committee and how it works, the procedures described as well as the makeup of the committee are representative of one kind of school. In a similar fashion the information in the profiles of the applicants is based on interviews at one school. Other schools will have their own standards, will seek their own goals, and will select students for their schools in their own way.

At some schools, especially state institutions, the emphasis is on producing primary care physicians who will provide service to the residents of the state. State schools have larger classes than private schools. A few of them have close to 300 students in each of the four classes. Private schools — that is, those that do not depend on the state for funds — can limit the size of their classes. State schools favor admission of applicants who are residents of the state. And the state legislature has something to say about the numbers of students admitted. Private schools talk about geographic diversity. Anyone can apply to a private school.

There will be differences between public and private institutions with regard to the philosophy of teaching and learning and, of course, in fees. However, the actual knowledge gained by the time the individual student receives the MD degree will, for practical purposes, be the same. What the graduate does with that knowledge is something else.

CHAPTER

1

The Admissions Committee And How It Works

M ost of the applicants are young people in their third year of college who will receive the degree of Bachelor of Arts or Bachelor of Science after four years of undergraduate study. Some who apply will get their bachelor's degree after three years of intensive undergraduate work that might include advanced placement credit for college-level courses taken in high school. A small number of applicants have the degree of Master of Arts or Doctor of Philosophy. There are students applying for the second or third time because of not having been accepted in previous years or because, after having been accepted in an earlier year, they decided to take a break in the academic routine and postpone matriculation in medical school. Some medical schools have programs in which the courses of study for the bachelor's degree and the medical degree are combined.

The Applications

Not all of the applications sent out are returned. At one medical school that filled approximately 9,000 individual requests for applications to enter the first year class of 1975-76, 2,943 were returned. The difference between the number of applications sent and those returned might be a result of one or several factors. The potential applicant might have decided upon a nonmedical career or might have changed his or her mind about an individual school after receiving the application and reading the requirements for admission or the average break-off point with regard to scores on the Medical College Admission Test and cumulative grade point averages. Applicants might not be interested in the rigidity or flexibility of the curriculum offered by a particular school. And some might be discouraged by the description in the school's prospectus of what is expected of the medical students. For example, a requirement for the award of the MD degree might include, in addition to the regular courses in basic science and clinical medicine, the completion of a thesis based upon research in laboratory, or investigation of a clinical problem or a field study of a community health project.

Screening

After the application is completed by the student and returned to the registrar, it is held until the results of the Medical College Admission Test and letters of recommendation arrive. The fully completed application is assigned for screening to members of the faculty who serve on the admissions committee. The process of screening is rotated with two people doing the job every week. Screening is done independently by each of the people to whom the application is assigned. Each of them reads the application and gives it a numerical rating based on its contents. Cumulative grade point averages as well as grades obtained in science courses, scores on the MCAT, descriptions of extracurricular activities, letters of recommendation from faculty members at the college at which the student carried out his or her undergraduate work and letters from employers are evaluated. Recommendations from personal friends of the applicant's family might not be as valuable as those from instructors and employers. If the application is given a high rating by each of the people who did the screening, the applicant will be invited to the school for a personal interview.

The Interview and Rating

The applicant has the option of accepting or declining the invitation. If the applicant proceeds with the interview at the medical school, he or she will have the opportunity to meet students at that school who can answer questions and supply information that the applicant might be interested in knowing. In addition, the applicant will meet at least one member of the faculty and perhaps two or more. Sometimes members of the admissions committee visit other schools to conduct regional interviews. Occasionally a graduate of the medical school who is not a member of the admissions committee but who lives near the applicant's college will interview the student on home ground so that the applicant does not have to travel a great distance. Often it is better to talk directly with a member of the admissions committee at the school to which one has applied.

Usually the applicant is interviewed by two people. The admissions committee meets regularly once a week. At that meeting the applicants interviewed the preceding week are presented in absentia by the interviewers. The members of the committee who have not interviewed the student listen and ask questions. They may challenge the interviewers' analyses, interpretations of the student's ability, motivation, achievements and so on. The interviewer has the opportunity to play the role of advocate for the applicant. The committee as a whole assigns the applicant to one of several categories such as *hold, probably accept* or *reject.*

At one medical school three marathon meetings are held during the academic year. At each of those meetings crucial decisions are made, and one-third of the class are selected. If both interviewers have given the student the highest rating, it is likely that the student will be accepted. It is also possible that a student with high ratings will not be accepted but will be put in a hold category if more applicants were rated *accept* than there were places for filling one-third of the class. If that were the case the applicant would be reconsidered at the next marathon meeting when the second third of the class would be accepted. If one interviewer has given a student a high rating while another has given the same student a low rating, an attempt to reach a compromise is made. The student might be held for reconsideration later in the year, or a third interview might be requested. Hence, the applicants who were interviewed and were not rejected at one of the weekly meetings can be considered for acceptance three times during the year.

2
The Members Of
The Committee

At one school, eighteen physicians recently served on the committee of admissions, three of whom were women. Sixteen were full-time members of the faculty receiving their salaries from their respective departments at the medical school or other divisions of the university. Two people had clinical appointments at the medical school with their income derived from private practice. There are no funds allotted for salaries for the physicians working on the committee. There is an auxiliary committee that interviews applicants when members of the regular committee are not available. They are helpful but their role is not great. The registrar of the school of medicine, a woman with heavy responsibility for the functioning of the committee, meets most of the applicants but does not interview them or vote on the committee. The active committee is small, busy, and hardworking.

The members of the committee on admissions are proposed by the steering committee of the Medical School Council, a group representing, in a very broad sense, various segments of the medical school — for example, tenured, nontenured, and part-time faculty; medical students; graduate students in public health; and members of the clinical house staff.

During a recent period the members of this committee were in the following specialties: anatomy, cell biology, dermatology, epidemiology, genetics, immunology, internal medicine, molecular biophysics and biochemistry, neurosurgery, obstetrics and gynecology, orthopedics, pediatrics, psychiatry, public health, radiobiology, and radiology. Two people had dual appointments and another person had three. Often there are members of the regular committee who hold the PhD degree and not the MD; some have both the MD and PhD degrees.

The Head of the Committee

A dispassionate scholar, he is productive in his field of specialization and is an indefatigable writer. Calm, cool, and composed, he listens to the presentations of the other interviewers, to both sides of the argument when there is one, and, in an even tone, quietly suggests a compromise. Indeed, compromise is the hallmark of decisions by committee. He interviews more applicants than any other member of the committee, tries to be fair, and does not become emotionally involved with individual applicants. He described one individual as "naive. . .has been accepted elsewhere and should go there." Although he is an investigator and not involved in patient-care, he, together with most of the members of the committee, looks for the potentially good doctor.

The Clinicians

The physicians involved in diagnosis and treatment of patients' illnesses, and who are full-time members of the faculty, also have responsibilities for teaching medical students and members of the hospital staff. Some of them carry out clinical research and, less commonly, laboratory research. All of them are concerned with getting smart applicants who will practice medicine. A few seek the medical scholar, someone who will add knowledge to the field or maintain a lifelong interest in acquiring knowledge for one's own sake in keeping up to date. Not many people look for academicians, and one or two are antiscience.

A clinician who is himself a productive scientist at a basic level referred to an applicant as "a man who knows science but is stiff and boardlike." The same day he interviewed the man who knows science he talked with, and was greatly impressed by, a young woman who was weak in the physical sciences but knowledgeable in psychology and who was an interesting conversationalist.

A clinician who is a genuine medical scholar, knowing his own field in depth and doing clinical research while remaining an admired teacher, looks for the intelligent applicant who has proved himself or herself in some endeavor. Whether this project was the major subject in college or a side interest, such as composing or performing music or writing a book, the physician, when impressed by an applicant, becomes so enthusiastic that he praises the individual with grandiloquence that increases mightily as successive applicants of excellence are seen. One lofty phrase follows another: "the best I have seen. . ." and "the most superb. . .a unique talent." Although the praise may be exaggerated, it is good to have a member of the committee who is strongly supportive of the highly qualified applicants rather than one who says, "Put the person on the waiting list — middle or low — whichever is empty."

A clinician in a surgical specialty who has a strong interest in mental health and counseling explained his negative reaction to an applicant with an outstanding scholastic record as an undergraduate in the college of the university at which he was being interviewed for a place in the first year class at the medical school. The student's cumulative grade point average was 3.67 and his percentile ratings in the Medical College Admission Test were all in the 90's except for one score in the 80's in the section on general information. He indicated that he had attended the college because his parents wanted him to go there and that he did not want to spend another four years in the same location. Then why did he apply? He figured that he might just as well toss his application on the pile. Perhaps that comment reflected the student's sense of humor. The interviewer believed, however, that applying to medical school is a serious step and the interview is a serious occasion.

Conclusion: one should not treat with unsuitable levity an occasion as serious as an interview for admission to medical school.

The Psychiatrists

Always interesting in their analyses of the candidates, they sometimes go into depth in their interviews. Their own interests in literature, music, art, and the theatre often surface such as in the comment by one impressed by an applicant with a European background: "the quintessential intellectual." Another candidate: "lively, refreshing, personable." Or simply "glib." The power of decision by a psychiatrist is significant when the interview is a bad one, for there is no recourse when the psychiatrist says "reject."

The Surgeons

They are often direct and not verbose, referring to applicants as "superficial, not impressive." And, "This person can do anything . . . I hope he goes into my specialty." Or, "She hasn't done anything in depth . . . a dilettante, a dabler."

The Scientists

There are three physicians who do work in basic science. Two of them hold PhD degrees as well as MD degrees and are top-notch investigators. The one without the PhD does research at a basic level and is also a clinical consultant in a medical specialty. All three are bright and perceptive. None of them makes a point of looking for a potential medical scientist. All are tuned in to looking for the good doctor.

The scientists' discussions of the people they have interviewed are not out of the ordinary. For example, with regard to an applicant with a cumulative grade point average of 3.8 and percentile scores of 83 and 99 in the mathematics and science sections on the MCAT, a scientist, responding to a surgeon's description of a candidate who had been interviewed by both, asked, "You say you didn't find anything unusual about him?" "Yes," came the answer. "Well," came the rejoinder, "I thought he was the worst candidate I have ever seen."

Another scientist discussed a *safe* candidate he had interviewed. "Every once in awhile he would ask me to repeat what I said. But I couldn't remember, either!"

Interviewers are supposed to make the applicants comfortable. It is likely that the applicant who makes the interviewer comfortable is on his or her way to success.

The Interviewers for the Minorities

Minorities are people who differ from the majority of the population. Minority applicants to medical school are considered to be those persons who differ from the majority of the applicants in being disadvantaged educationally, economically, and, perhaps, culturally. The category of cultural deprivation might be in the mind of the arrogant beholder. In practice, members of minorities are people with a significant amount of the pigment melanin in their skin. They include the following groups: Black Americans, Native Americans, Asian Americans, people with Spanish surnames (from the Island of Puerto Rico and the mainland of North America), and Mexican Americans.

Economically and educationally deprived white people are neither sought nor welcomed as members of a disadvantaged group when committees on admissions to medical schools are sitting. It is possible that people refuse to believe that there is such an entity as the disadvantaged white person in North America although the evidence is stunning. It is easy to think that people with darkly pigmented skin are the only disadvantaged group because the majority of North Americans in the professions have lightly pigmented skin, whereas people with dark skin are underrepresented in the professions.

Every applicant from a minority group is interviewed by a person on the admissions committee who is also a member of a minority group and, when possible, by a second member of the committee who is not part of a minority. It is desirable for all applicants to medical school who have survived the screening process to be interviewed by two people.

Of the three members on the admissions committee who regularly interview applicants from minority groups, as well as applicants who are not part of a minority, two are North American blacks and one is an Asian American. Two are full-time members of the faculty with professorial rank and one is in full-time practice in the community. These individuals are smart, quick-witted, and favored with the gift of verbal agility. Not only are their comments instructive and fun to listen to, but, more important, they have a keen understanding of the applicants—and their opinions are respected.

The fun and the reality: "Hooray! I really found this application exciting; I liked the applicant." Or, "Very bright, very young, and very arrogant — reject!" In an exchange between an interviewer who is a member of a minority group and another who is not but who interviewed the same applicant, feelings ran deep. The interviewer who is not a member of a minority said, with no little exasperation, that the applicant should not be accepted because he had not had any exposure to clinical medicine and that the only thing he had going for him was his interest and high ability in math. The quick but gentle rejoinder from the minority member of the committee was that minority people with that talent are rare and desirable. The applicant was accepted but decided to go to another school.

Random Pickings Gleaned at a Meeting

An attractive, bright, and pleasant woman who earned straight A's in her last semester at a college to which she had transferred from another school, where she had not done so well, was excellent in basic research and asked her interviewer if she could get a job in his laboratory. He had recognized her ability and offered her a job on the spot. Another applicant who had a PhD in one of the hard sciences but was interested in becoming a physician was tossed aside by one interviewer as having "pre-tenure anxiety."

An interviewer not noted for personal warmth described an applicant as "brusque, cold, and distant." Another physician complimented another student: "He is a nuclear generator of intellectual activity." A third, discussing a third applicant, said "he scared the shit out of me!" A pediatrician and an internist vis-á-vis the same applicant: "not diffuse"; and "diffuse, I say!"

Some candidates are described as being *safe*, the translation of which is not outstanding. A *solid* candidate will make the grade; a *ho-hum* applicant is neither safe nor solid.

The End of the Marathon

At the last meeting of the academic year, champagne is served. Everybody hopes that the applicants who were accepted will accept the invitation to come to the school.

CHAPTER **3**

The Applicants:
50 Case Studies

A comparison of applicants who were successful in gaining admission to medical school and those who were not might enable a prospective student to draw conclusions that would be helpful in an interview. Fifty students who were interviewed for admission to the entering class at one medical school are described.

1. Our first candidate is a 22-year-old woman who, because of her wit, independence, and glamour, could tame Petruchio. At the age of 16, having skipped the senior year of high school, she was granted early admission to an outstanding university in the Midwest. After the first quarter's work, during which she earned an A in calculus and B's in biophysics, humanities, and social science, she transferred to a college in the city where her family lived. There she maintained an almost straight A average with a major in chemistry and a strong background in mathematics, physics, French, Russian, and assorted courses in English, economics, classical and western civilization, and psychology.

There was a 15-month hiatus in her academic work because of the death by suicide of her father followed not long after by the death of her mother who had hypertension and cardiac disease. When the applicant left college after her father's death, she went to live with her mother who became emotionally dependent upon her. The daughter recognized that responsibility for the care of a young sibling had become hers and not her mother's. After the mother's death, the youngster went to live with a relative in another part of the country and the applicant was able to go it alone. Not only did she complete college while doing clerical work on weekends at a large medical center, but she was graduated with the degree of Bachelor of Science, summa cum laude, and was a member of Phi Beta Kappa.

Her science grade point average was 3.9 and her cumulative grade point average was 3.8. Her percentile scores on the Medical College Admission Test were verbal 94, quantitative 97, general information 95, and science 98. Although the background she gained in science while in college would enable her to pursue a career in research, her preference is to deal with people on a one-to-one basis as a physician.

Her extracurricular activities in college included membership in a language club and a hiking group and taking part in a National Science Foundation summer research program. Among the things she has enjoyed most were studying quantum mechanics and traveling in Europe, especially in Rome, because of her interest in archeology. After being graduated from college, she found it necessary to take a year off in order to establish a firm financial base since competition for financial aid in medical school is vigorous.

Letters of recommendation from her instructors were excellent and included such statements as the following: biology: "the most outstanding student I have instructed in my five years at College"; physics: "was my best student. . .must rank in the top one or two percent overall of [pre-meds] at least as far as physics is concerned"; chemistry: "unusually well motivated and intelligent. . .has a stable and compassionate personality"; mathematics: "her work showed originality and insight"; economics: "the best of 80 students."

Was she accepted? One interviewer gave her a high rating for acceptance. The other interviewer, visibly disturbed, gave her a low rating because she had not had any direct medical experience in a hospital setting — and how did she know that she really wanted to go into medicine? The first interviewer felt that the applicant had unusually high ability, impeccable credentials, and strong motivation for a career in medicine. The second interviewer was turned off by the background in theoretical science. The discussion at the meeting of the admissions committee increased in warmth as the arguments were tossed back and forth. The head of the committee announced that there would be a break in the meeting during which the two interviewers could try to resolve their differences and come to an amicable solution. The interviewer who had pushed for the applicant's acceptance left the handsome wood-paneled room in search of a cigarette. Upon return that interviewer was told not to worry, things would get worked out. The result? The student was not accepted immediately but was accepted midway in the academic year. She declined the acceptance, having made a decision to go to another school that had accepted her earlier. It would not be fair to infer that the student enrolled in the other school simply because she had been accepted there first. The explanation she gave was "for personal reasons." Later it was learned that she had married, and it was better for her husband's career that they live in another city.

2. Lorenzo Leibniz is a 20-year-old applicant for the Medical Scientist Training Program — affectionately dubbed "Mud-Phud" — a plan that enables the student to pursue a course of study leading to both an MD and a PhD degree after six years of work. He is the kind of young man the interviewer would like to have as a classmate in medical school: he seems to be a nice person. Bright, serious, and pleasant, he wants to acquire knowledge for himself, for doing investigative work, and for helping people. There is no question about his strength of purpose in wanting to do research in molecular biophysics and biochemistry with a medical basis. He is dedicated to a career in an academic setting with some association with clinical problems. His brother is a third-year medical student at another school. His mother is a social worker and his father is a dentist.

Mr. Leibniz, who did not go to either of the universities attended by his parents, was graduated from a small college for men with a Bachelor of Science degree, with honors in chemistry and philosophy. In addition to the numerous courses in the subjects of his major, there were several in mathematics and physics and others in English and French literature, psychology, and economics. Both his science grade point average and cumulative grade point average were 3.9. His percentile ratings in the MCAT were verbal 96, quantitative 99, general information 83, and science 98.

His extracurricular activities included work as a laboratory instructor in physical chemistry, membership on the varsity team in lacrosse, computer programming for the chemistry department, serving as president for his dormitory and as a campus guide, directing a bridge club — he is a national master in the American Contract Bridge League — and teaching life saving for the American Red Cross. He did research in biochemistry and pharmacology during the summers before his sophomore, junior, and senior years.

Mr. Leibniz's letters of recommendation were superb and included the following remarks: chemistry "a joy to have in class because he becomes actively involved"; biology: "thoughtful and creative . . . almost like a colleague rather than a student"; philosophy: "one of the most imaginative and analytical students"; Committee on recommendations: "one of our *very* top students."

Although he had been accepted by two excellent schools, one in the North and one in the South, he is interested in the school at which he is being interviewed because the course setup is flexible so that obtaining the MD and PhD degrees simultaneously will not be a hassle. Also, he believes that competition will be less of a problem than it is at another school attended by his best friend, a first year medical student, who complains that the pressure of exams and jockeying for grades are enervating.

Mr. Leibniz is a superior candidate who, among applicants to medical school, would be considered a "gasper," a colloquial synonym for superstar. The people who interviewed Mr. Leibniz for the medical school and the graduate school wanted him in their programs. He accepted the invitation.

3. Corky Dillon is a 21-year-old red-haired woman with a sunny disposition who will be graduated with the degrees of Bachelor of Arts in biology and Master of Science in medical genetics from a small but good university. She is a chatterbox who bubbles with enthusiasm. Ms. Dillon is interested in medical genetics from all standpoints but particularly diagnosis, treatment, and prevention in order to counsel families who are suffering from the burden of transmission of an abnormal gene. She believes that the counselor should be as well trained in the laboratory as in the clinic to be able to decide whether a problem is caused by a mutation, a chromosomal abnormality, or a biochemical defect.

To become knowledgeable and confident and also to satisfy her innate curiosity, she applied to the combined MD-PhD program with the intention of doing further graduate study in the department of human genetics. However, sometime after the date on which she filed her application and before discussion with the second interviewer, her ardor for the PhD degree cooled while her desire to do genetic counseling expanded. Part of her seeming change in goals might be a realization that basically she is not keen on the intensity and dedication required for the PhD; part might reflect her pleasure in talking with the first interviewer — an excellent clinical geneticist — who introduced her to the possibility of acquiring training for genetic counseling through the mechanism of a fellowship after completing the requirements for an MD degree.

Ms. Dillon's enthusiasm is boundless and extended to singing in musical groups in college, as well as with a chorous that accompanied the notable symphony orchestra in her hometown, voluntary tutoring enthusiastic and included the following comments. From the premedical advisory committee: "Corky Dillon is an absolutely outstanding visiting the adult correction center once a week and talking with the prisoners.

She worked each summer in learning types of jobs. For example, in the summer before her first year at college she worked as a laboratory assistant at a university near her home examining the effect of radiation on the mitotic cycle of a mold. The summer following her first year she got a secretarial job in a private hospital and volunteered her services in a laboratory of endocrinology and metabolism where she learned the technique of tissue culture of cells from tumors. She had no difficulty obtaining a job, a high-paying one, in a hemodialysis unit during the second summer by writing a physician at the suggestion of a classmate. Not only did she learn about kidney function and make more money than the regular employees in the hospital but, best of all, the hospital was located in a European country that American students take special delight in visiting.

Ms. Dillon does not lack get-up-and-go. Before the summer following her third year of college she had read a testbook on genetics written by a physician at a hospital in the Middle East. She simply wrote him a letter, based on her familiarity with his book, and got the opportunity to take part in a study on a genetic disorder and also do library research abroad.

If Ms. Dillon had sufficient time, she would live in different environments and absorb different languages. She made clear that she has no intention of jumping around to other countries while in medical school. Although this young woman is not reticent, one must not make the mistake of thinking she is superficial. She is bright and a serious thinker who wants to know enough cytogenetics and biochemistry to understand clinical problems in genetics.

This lively young woman, whose father is a school counselor and whose mother is a social worker, earned a science and a cumulative grade point average of 3.8. Her numerous recommendations were in chemistry and mathematics, grading math papers, serving as a teaching assistant in microbiology, playing intramural sports, and prospect for medical school, very promising as a candidate for the MD-PhD degrees''; chemistry first year: ''the best of several hundred students. . .as close to an ideal student as one could hope for. . .the kind of pest I like to have around''; organic chemistry: ''this year's highest (gold-plated) recommendation''; physical chemistry: ''first rate''; history: ''thoughtful and provocative reports''; mathematics: ''her final examination was first and far from number two.''

Not all the remarks were laudatory; some had an edge of criticism: French literature: ''passive in class. . .little ability to develop ideas''; religious studies: ''I graded her work as B. . .but it was the highest of the B's. . .perhaps [quality of participation] influenced by [student's] priorities.''

Ms. Dillon was accepted. She withdrew after receiving her acceptance to another school in a different part of the country.

4. Ramon Morales is a neatly dressed 19-year-old, self-confident person with the pink cheeks characteristic of the teenager being treated with topical agents for acne. His family consists of his father, an author, his mother, a professor of Spanish-American literature, and an older brother who is a physician married to a physician. Young Morales, who was born in Cuba, will reach 20 soon after he completes his third and last year at college with a major in mathematics. He expects to be elected to Phi Beta Kappa and to receive a Bachelor of Science degree, summa cum laude, with a major in mathematics.

Mr. Morales speaks with ease and affability. He is bright as well as articulate and projects himself into the future as an academician who teaches, takes care of patients, and does research. How does he know about research? He did a laboratory study on the effect of specific substances on aging in fruit flies. The research had been tedious, he said, and he would not object to having other people do research under his direction. When questioned about the wisdom of that approach to getting something done, he answered that perhaps one must do it oneself. He has been geared toward medicine since high school and feels that the requirement of a thesis is a good one because it gives a student the chance to explore research and do something original. His declared hope is to balance clinical practice with postdoctoral study, research, and teaching.

The applicant's grades were superior. He had taken several courses in mathematics, the minimum in chemistry and physics that would be acceptable for admission to medical school, and a reasonable number in biology, the social sciences, and the humanities. His science and cumulative grade point averages were 3.9 and his percentile ratings on the MCAT were verbal 94, quantitative 70, general information 98, and science 93. Because the quantitative score seemed low for a student of mathematics and because many applicants have said that the quantitative test reflects knowledge of high school rather than of college math and also measures skill in performing rapid calculations, it seemed worthwhile to look at his transcript from high school.

He had scored 99 percent in the National Educational Development Test given in 10th grade, 97 percent in the Practice Scholastic Aptitude Test and in the 700s in the Scholastic Aptitude Test. Ordinarily, one does not look at the high school rating of an applicant to medical school because that transcript is not included in the application to medical school, nor should it be. In the case of Mr. Morales, comparing the result in the MCAT to that in other tests was helpful.

Extracurricular activities included membership in Spanish and mathematics clubs, a literary group, and an experimental theatre. He had been employed by the department of mathematics as a tutor and worked voluntarily for the American Red Cross. The summers before and during college had been spent taking courses and traveling in North America, Europe, and Africa.

One letter of recommendation came, and that was from the committee on recommendations from Mr. Morales's college. It was enthusiastic and strongly supportive for a student whom they considered an unusual candidate from their school.

Mr. Morales is smart, capable, determined, and immature. The good characteristics outweigh the last one. He was not accepted immediately although his credentials were excellent. It is possible, although not certain, that he let one of the people on the admissions committee who interviews minority applicants know that he did not want to be considered for admission as a member of a minority group. That explanation is speculative. Mr. Morales was placed on the waiting list and was accepted — as a candidate from a minority group.

5. Becky Stein is a neatly dressed 23-year-old college graduate. She has little poise, no equanimity, and may feel like the rabbit facing the stoat. Nevertheless, the interview is an interesting one for the interviewer. And perhaps for the interviewee? She is serious, quiet, shy, and not polished or articulate; that is, she is hesitant in verbalizing her thoughts. But when she does, they are vigorously effective.

Ms. Stein had majored in biology at a highly competitive urban university with an open admissions policy. Her interest in biology had been strong enough to think about getting a PhD at one time, but no more. In order to get away from the city one summer, and away from the family's inadequate apartment in a dangerous neighborhood, she enrolled in a graduate program in biology at a university in the Southwest. This intelligent and honest girl recognized that false start for what it was. She did not want to do research; she wanted to be a physician. There is no doubt that admission to medical school would be a fulfillment of a long-standing dream. She believes that her background will enable her to bring both understanding and compassion into the medical profession. That background is one of poverty and social and educational deprivation. Her parents had been in concentration camps in the early 1940s, and after they came to the

United States, before the applicant was born, the father — described as a laborer — was unable to work. He died of a myocardial infarct during Ms. Stein's sophomore year at college. She withdrew from school for a while in order to work in a store and help support the family. The mother has a poorly paying job as a cook in a home for the aged. There are two siblings, one in college and one in high school. The family is on welfare.

Ms. Stein's strongest work in college was in the humanities, especially in creative writing for which she had won cash prizes in short story contests. Several pieces of her fiction recently appeared in highly respected journals. Her professor of English wrote that she was one of the brightest students he had had the good fortune to teach as well as being the best writer and the hardest worker. A novelist, in whose creative writing course she worked last year, described her as incredibly intelligent, a person who really cares about being a doctor and who has remarkable emotional stability considering her terrible background. In addition to serving as a volunteer in a hospital and working in a biochemistry laboratory for four months, she worked for two summers in the greenhouse of a botanical garden reorganizing a seed collection, grafting, and repotting exotic plants. One of the experiences she enjoyed most was taking part in a survival course in a wilderness area in the mountains of Oregon.

Her cumulative grade point average was 3.3 and her science grade point average was 3.1. She completed the premedical science requirements with more B's than A's or C's. Her scores in the MCAT were poor the first time around and rose to a respectable level in the tests for verbal ability, 83, and general information, 98, when repeated. Her performance in the quantitative, 23, and scientific, 54, sections remained lower than the averages attained by most of the students attending the medical school to which she had applied but was similar to those of other applicants from a disadvantaged background.

Although Ms. Stein likes writing and is good at it, her hope, wish, and great desire is to be a physician taking care of patients but not on a private fee-for-service basis. Of the several medical schools to which she applied, she was invited for interviews at four prestigious ones. She was not accepted by any. Nor was she considered a member of a disadvantaged group although socially, educationally, and economically she is imprisoned in that group. She is considered a high risk because of her poor testing ability.

The first interviewer was willing to take that risk because of the applicant's keen intelligence, strong motivation to become a physician, and ability to begin a project and follow it through to completion as proved by her creative writing. A second interviewer tossed her off as a poet whom he could not see as a physician. A third interviewer with much experience thought the applicant's ideas about medicine were unrealistic but made some positive suggestions: study additional courses in science, get her hands dirty in hospital work, repeat the MCAT, and apply to medical school another year.

The applicant is not depressed but she is worried. Her self-confidence is not great. She wants to know: "If I do these things, will it really make a difference?" It did not. She reapplied the following year and again was rejected.

6. The ambassador's daughter is a study in grace. Her every movement, from seating herself to lifting her hands in reaction to a question or to complement an answer, suggests the quiet but purposeful elegance of the trained dancer. Her maturity makes her seem older, in a positive way, than her 23 years. Although she is outwardly composed, intense concern about being admitted to medical school is much in evidence. She is worried.

Ms. Josephine Frederick had been graduated from a *lycée* in Paris and is now, six years later, completing work toward a Bachelor of Arts degree in biology at a university in the United States. Her grades in biology, physics, calculus, advanced chemistry, and all the humanities are straight A's with outstanding recommendations. Her percentile scores in the MCAT represent an interesting phenomenon. The first time she took the examination, four years after being out of school and without much background in the sciences, the verbal was 94, quantitative 77, general information 86, and science 21. The second time around the verbal remained high, quantitative dropped 16 points, general information fell 33 points, and science rose to 41. The third and last time her scores were verbal 97, quantitative 98, general information 91, and science 98. She is embarrassed about taking the MCAT three times but did so because she is determined to go into medicine. She feels that she has gone in enough different directions to have worked things out thoroughly before making that career choice.

Among her studies were the languages of Sanskrit, Tamil, and Tibetan, and Hindu and Buddhist philosophy and the Indian theory of aesthetics. During her ten years in India she had learned one of the classical Indian temple dances and had given solo performances in India, Nepal, and Sri Lanka. She has put her knowledge of yoga — acquired in her training for the dance — to work in helping asthmatic patients who require exercises in breathing and other kinds of physical therapy.

Ms. Fredrick's father had attended college in another country and was an ambassador from that country. Her mother had been graduated from a fine college for women in the United States, and, although she had not acquired professional training, she managed to steal time from her duties as the wife of an ambassador to pursue scholarly interests in art, archeology, and other subjects encountered in the course of the family's travels and also to become an author. One brother was an architect and another was an economist. Both grandfathers were physicians, one a professor in a medical school and the other a clinical specialist. An uncle was a physician with a major interest in one medical disorder and had written a book on that topic. The doctor-author uncle had actively and successfully discouraged both his daughters from going into medicine — because they would only get married anyway — and had followed the same tack with his niece from her thirteenth year to the present. Ms. Fredrick reflected, with bitterness sweetened by compassion, that her two cousins were in their thirties with no marital ties and regretted their not going into medicine.

The applicant wants to go into medical practice, possibly cardiology. There is no doubt that she will be an excellent physician. She was not given an immediate acceptance because of the crush of good applicants but was put in a very high position on the waiting list. A letter was sent asking her if she wanted to be on the waiting list. There was no answer. Checking the records of the American Medical College Application Service disclosed that Ms. Fredrick had been accepted by, and had accepted admission to, a large medical school in a large city.

7. The interviewer was surprised but not disappointed to meet Bradford Burns. As all Americans know, except perhaps interviewers, one cannot distinguish ethnic groups simply by name and often not by appearance. In the United States English and Scottish first names and last names can belong to an Asian American as rightfully as to a descendant of forebears from the British Isles.

Mr. Burns is a wide awake, straightforward, nonhesitant, interesting 20-year-old who is hooked on independence. His father is dead. Although he has a half brother, a pediatrician who works in a prepaid medical service in another part of the state in which they live, he is for practical purposes an only child because 20 years separate him and his sibling. His mother is dependent on young Mr. Burns and he has been trying to wean himself away. Their livelihood is based on a take-out food business. Mr. Burns helps in the financial management.

In the summer before his final year in high school, Mr. Burns attended a state university not far from home in order to get the experience of being in college. In the fall, while in high school, he also attended college, a city one, because he had only four courses to complete in high school. He was trying, little by little, to leave home.

The following year he matriculated at a college where he studied for four years and obtained a Bachelor of Arts degree with a combined major in chemistry and zoology. His program included difficult courses in addition to those required of premedical students and he achieved a cumulative grade point average of 3.8 and a science grade point average of 3.9. On the MCAT his percentile ratings were verbal 92, quantitative 97, general information 87, and science 99. He had been a laboratory assistant in biochemistry, a student representative on the college council, a member of the dormitory council, and a student advisor for freshmen. He also had been a member of the faculty evaluation committee but there was nothing to do because no one came up for tenure consideration in the natural sciences at that time. Further activities included hiking in the Sierras, repairing his car, and studying Mandarin. He already knew Cantonese.

He spent three summers in funded research that included one clinical project and two in the basic sciences. He is knowledgeable about all aspects of the research. The clinical study represented a good idea but was not successful. One of the projects in basic science involved a difficult procedure of synthesis and neither the student nor his advisors got it to work. He also worked at a hospital where he helped with cardiac catheterization, observed surgical procedures, and attended conferences and made ward rounds.

Mr. Burns believes that medicine combines scientific investigation with the opportunity to work with people. The potential range of working — from being a medical scientist to being a family practitioner — seems to be an ideal compromise. However, he is not really interested in research. He recognizes that it requires time, patience, and perseverance. One thing he knows: he does not want to be at someone else's mercy. His choices within the broad field of medicine are wide open and he would not hazard a guess about a specific choice. At the end of an interesting interview he said, "I can even see myself as a Beverly Hills physician!" The interviewer can hardly wait to see what happens four years hence.

8. Jean Kaler, neat in appearance and pleasant of personality, with a way of thinking that could be described as precise but not prim, is a high school teacher of mathematics who, because of her vast age of 26 years, speaks of herself as the older woman trying to get into medical school. She earned a Bachelor of Arts degree, magna cum laude, at a midwestern university accumulating a grade point average of 3.7 and a science average of 3.9. She had been elected to Phi Beta Kappa and was a member of Mortar Board, the student senate, and the hockey club, and had worked as an assistant in the mathematics department.

While in high school she had thought about a career in medicine and had served as a candy striper. Her parents, both teachers in public schools, had nourished the medical interests of their older child, a son, but not those of their daughter. The son became a general practitioner and the daughter set out on a career in education, obtaining the degree of Master of Arts in Teaching. She felt that becoming a high school teacher would allow her to work with and help people — the latter being what she considered her primary goal in medicine — but medicine as a career was not as reachable as teaching. Nevertheless, during her first two years in college she had studied, in addition to the humanities, zoology, general chemistry, and quantitative analysis but not organic chemistry. The though of medicine had not left her.

She went on to teach in two eastern cities, two of the high schools being the type that sends many students to college and one being in a disadvantaged area from which few students go on to college. On the basis of these experiences in teaching and her recollections, as well as those of her colleagues, of students' attitudes and behavior at the time she had been in high school, she had made some interesting observations about high school teaching and high school students. She believes that in the most recent years of her teaching the students have become more passive and less excited about school work and even extracurricular activities. She does not believe there is a significant difference in interest and excitement between students at the more academic secondary schools and those attending schools in deprived neighborhoods. In one highly thought of school in a small college town in the East, in proximity to several universities, the students would sit in class and wait for the bell to ring. They would be glad to get back to school after vacation and they couldn't wait until vacation time came around again. The easy opportunity to ski, sail, travel, or work on a project was greeted with no more anticipation than the dread of finding or not finding a job.

Ms. Kaler feels that there is a great difference in students' interests today and the level of interest ten years ago. She sees little or no creativity or unique accomplishments, with but rare exceptions. How does she identify creativity? She looks for interest in a particular subject, artistic or scientific endeavor, how the student occupies time, what he or she does from 3 o'clock on. Something out of the ordinary would stand out. She thinks one can spot *lack* of creativity, for example, in people who just go along with the crowd. Does she have any suggestions about the cause of the inertia she describes? Television, perhaps, because the box promotes a passive existence.

Ms. Kaler is married to a man whose major interest is writing poetry. Her major interest is in family practice. She could not be a scientist; she does not have the interest or the personality required for investigative work. She wants to provide health care for people who cannot get it because of financial, social, or geographic factors.

This woman, with an uncommon amount of common sense, was not accepted outright by any of the medical schools to which she applied. Her performance on the MCAT might have had something to do with her rejections. Her percentile scores were verbal 77, quantitative 95, general information 67, and science 17. The MCAT had been taken before the applicant had studied organic chemistry. The suggestion was made that she repeat the test. She did and raised her score. Still there were no acceptances. Almost a year after submitting her application she received a call from the registrar at one medical school inviting her to join the entering class in the fall. There was a pause, and then Ms. Kaler's response, "Is this for real?" Applicant and registrar were delighted.

9. Henry Helmholtz is a funny, serious, agile, nonathletic, Talmudic-like irreligionist. A coiner of words, singer of phrases with an upward lilt, mathematical wizard, physicist-chemist, enthusiastic, future scholar-investigator, he seeks admittance to the Medical Scientist Training Program. The challenge is not for him to gain acceptance to a medical school but for the medical school to woo, entice, and proselytize, if necessary, to win the candidate.

Mr. Helmholtz had been admitted to college with sophomore standing on the basis of high scores on advanced placement examinations in six subjects: American and European history, English, calculus, chemistry, and physics. As an undergraduate, he had achieved the highest score nationally in the year in which he took part in the Society of Actuaries mathematical competition.

By the end of his four years at college he would collect a Bachelor of Arts degree with a combined major in chemistry and physics and a Master of Arts degree in chemistry. His undergraduate work included courses in the humanities, history, government, the social sciences, and expository writing in addition to biology, chemistry, and physics. His cumulative and science grade point averages were over 3.9 — he had received a B+ in a course in government. He had been elected to Phi Beta Kappa in his junior year. His percentile scores on the MCAT were verbal 95, quantitative 97, general information 99, and science 98.

During three summers he worked in different laboratories in or near his hometown, read, and engaged in recreational sports. Extracurricular activities during the school year included taking part in daily discussions on science and logic and teaching a laboratory section in physics. His participation in extracurricular activities would be considered small when compared with the listings compiled by most applicants to medical school. He is honest about his interests and ambitions. In his own words, he has sampled both sides of the interface between medical research and practice and wants a combined career in both disciplines. Because he recognizes the need to be trained at the highest levels in order to understand human biology and identify new areas of interest relative to research and to medical practice, he is seeking a program leading to the MD and the PhD in molecular biophysics and biochemistry.

His recommendations soared above the usually glowing hyperbole routinely invoked by his university in describing their more earthly applicants to medical school: ''a phenomenal academic record. . .in a class by himself. . .a brilliant physicist. . .probably the top student in his class. . .young man who applies his prodigious abilities to human relations as well as to course work. . .has developed a solid circle of friends.'' The most joy-provoking comment was ''one problem is that he is on the inarticulate side. . .has made a real effort to improve his ability to communicate'' as opposed to ''very outgoing and always cheerful.''

Well, how is one to capture this candidate? Offer him money? That hypothetical suggestion is not as crass as it seems. The cost of a medical education, with or without pursuit of the PhD degree, is great, and most students require financial aid. Money would be the quickest answer, but it is in short supply because of the decrease in funds available from the federal government for the Medical Scientist Training Program.

Perhaps Mr. Helmholtz would be interested in meeting some of the people working in the labs on problems of medical significance? He would be and did. He himself suggested a young, full professor whom he would like to meet in addition to the members of the faculty to be encountered during the interview. No sooner asked than arranged. All went well. His being accepted by the admissions committee at the time of their next formal meeting was inevitable. But would he accept the school?

Gnawing at our hope was the knowledge that he had been offered a generous fellowship by a department at the university where he was completing his studies. The funds would be given, no strings attached, simply for his working in their laboratories during the summers of his tenure in medical school on a project of his choosing in the anticipation that he would make a discovery. No strings? Wasn't pressure to perform a rigorous fiber? No restriction on one's activities? The decision he had to make, although not accompanied by the kind of stress endured by the applicant who does not know whether he will get into any medical school, was an important one.

Perhaps he could gain some insight into what would be the best choice for himself by talking to students who had been in the MD-PhD program for a few years and also to people who had studied, worked, taught, done research, and practiced medicine at both the medical schools he was juggling? The personal investigations he made helped him to reach a decision: the combination of independence and the intellectual resources of the MD-PhD program at one school were compelling.

We were delighted to learn that we would be able to watch the development of a medical scholar.

10. Margaret Nova is a 20-year-old petite woman with curly hair who comes across as an alert, confident, friendly person. She is applying for the combined MD-PhD program. By dint of work and gift of brain she completed her studies for a Bachelor of Science degree with a major in biology in less than three years at a coeducational but predominantly male institution. In truth she had accumulated enough credits to be graduated after her second year because of having taken 16 courses, not easy ones, during the first year. The school's policy was that first year courses would be graded on a pass/fail basis. Ms. Nova had registered for a large number of courses because they seemed interesting, with the intention of dropping some after reaching a decision as to which would be most useful. She found, however, that it was not necessary to drop any; as indicated in letters from several instructors, had letter-grades been assigned, most of hers would have been A's.

Ms. Nova had decided to remain in college for a third year in order to study additional subjects, seize the opportunity to do research in biology, and take part in the nonacademic aspects of undergraduate life such as membership in a service fraternity of which she had become the president. Her courses included, in addition to a large number in biology and the required premedical subjects, mathematics, anthropology, psychology, philosophy, contemporary issues, art, and German. Her cumulative grade point average was 3.9 and her science grade point average was 3.8. Her percentile scores on the MCAT were verbal 97, quantitative 96, general information 95, and science 96.

Her extracurricular activities consisted largely of involvement with the service fraternity, being in charge of accounts for the school paper, and working as a teaching assistant in biology. Because her experience in teaching was pleasant, was financially profitable, and gave her more freedom than being a full-time student — in addition to providing a breathing space before beginning the next half-dozen years of schooling — she dropped the research project. Perhaps she would not do research. During the two summers following her first and second years of undergraduate study she held jobs, once for a company that packaged materials for use in scientific research and once in a private hospital. She also traveled in Europe.

Ms. Nova's family is from the Midwest, her father is a physician, her mother a teacher. She is one of five siblings, four of whom completed college with the fifth still in public school.

This bright and capable young woman, especially interested at present in problems relating to the storage of and access to memory, plans to get her PhD in molecular biophysics and biochemistry. Her excellent letters of recommendation can be summed up in one quotation: ''The world is her oyster.'' Her aim is to combine medical practice with research. She does not see herself in private practice but as a member of a hospital staff, a university, or in group practice.

She stated that the university at which she was being interviewed held more interest for her than all others, including the one at which she did her undergraduate work. She considered the latter restrictive because of its traditional emphasis on science and the obstacles imposed against working toward a PhD degree while enrolled in the medical school. Why did she prefer this university? Because of the good medical and graduate schools and the interaction between them. She liked the flexibility in the last one-and-a-half years of the medical curriculum and the opportunity to study molecular biophysics and biochemistry per se or to use its techniques to look for answers to questions originating at a macroscopic level.

Because of the applicant's enjoyment of teaching and service work and her small experience in research, and perhaps her plans to marry soon, the interviewer thought that the applicant's chief activity would be in clinical care rather than in academic research. Before the student left, the interviewer asked her a question commonly asked interviewees so that they can get back to home or to college easily: ''What can I do to help?'' The applicant answered sprightly, ''Get me into this medical school!''

Ms. Nova was accepted. She declined after notification that she had been moved up from her position on the waiting list to an acceptance category at the school at which she had done her undergraduate work.

11. Jeremy Galen is a wide-awake, neatly groomed 22-year-old. He was graduated from a relatively small, private eastern university that is known for the quality of its teaching in biology, music, and premedical studies. He majored in chemistry and accumulated a grade point average of 3.65. His college transcript was notable for the nonroutine, difficult science courses he had taken. His percentile scores in the MCAT ranged from a low of 97 to a high of 98. At the present time he is employed as a laboratory assistant at a state university helping to characterize the chemical and physical properties of enzymes. He does not particularly like the work he is doing but does it because he wants to be involved with something different from the academic work of the previous four years, because he wants to be in the environment of a medical school, and because he wants a job that pays more than the one available in a pulmonary function unit that might have been more interesting but was less profitable financially. During three of his years in college he held part-time jobs grading papers in mathematics four hours a week and working as a teller in a bank during vacations.

Although Mr. Galen's performance in science courses had been strong and he had been elected to Sigma Xi, his statements about not wanting a career in science are equally strong. To him science is simply a means of understanding medicine. He does not want to do laboratory work: he wants to do medical work: that is, work with people. And knowledge of science will help him become a better doctor. He does not want to use his scientific know-how to discover etiologic mechanisms of disease but does want to be a good diagnostician, maybe a medical scholar, but not an investigator. It is clear that Mr. Galen is not interested in research. He would favor buying dialysis machines for treatment of kidney disease over personally doing investigative work that might lead to measures that would prevent the disease and obviate the need for mechanical aids. Perhaps someone in college told him that if he took hard science courses he would be a better doctor.

Extracurricular activities included voluntary tutoring of high school students and serving as a member of the stage crew at a suburban youth theatre in his hometown. He wanted to act in the shows but all of them had been musicals and he could not sing. He had worked on the college daily paper but did not like writing. The association with the paper gave him an opportunity to meet people. He had been a section leader, helping to lead discussions in a group of ten students taking part in a course in human sexuality modeled after the course taught at the university at which he was being interviewed. One of the most interesting things he had done was to take a course in European history.

In his recommendations Mr. Galen was described as a solid prospect, not markedly outgoing but pleasant, intelligent, analytical, and conscientious. As a candidate for medical school he is smart, ambitious, and hardworking. He wants to be a good doctor and he is fully capable of becoming one. He was offered a place on the waiting list. Within a short time he was accepted into the medical school. The interviewer saw him again soon after matriculation. He said, "Remember, I'm not going to do research!"

> She sat with aplomb,
> Cooly calm.
> Medical College Aptitude Test,
> Grade point average among the best,
> No way could she bomb.

12. Nancy Sabin is a 21-year-old biology major who is neatly dressed, pleasant, and not at all tense as she relaxes in a chair opposite the interviewer. Neither enthusiastic nor apathetic, she seems accustomed to interviews. She had transferred to an Ivy League school after one year of study at a less prestigious university in the same area. Ms. Sabin, unlike the majority of women applying to medical school, is a candidate for the MD-PhD program. Her declared goal is to have a career combining research and clinical care.

Since high school she has done laboratory research during the summers — in hematology, genetics, and endocrinology — and is knowledgeable about all the projects on which she has worked. Extracurricular activities included serving on committees in her dormitory, helping to organize seminars, and tutoring one to three hours per week, more often before examination periods. With the money she earned from tutoring, she was able to take music lessons and learned to play the flute. She says that she has written short stories but has not submitted any for publication. Although working in a lab has been more interesting than anything else, she would not be satisfied unless she were treating patients. Her cumulative grade point average was 3.6 and her science grade point average was 3.5. Her scores on the MCAT were in the 90th percentile except for that in general information. Ms. Sabin was accepted into the MD-PhD program.

Nineteen days before the first year class was to register, Ms. Sabin wrote that she wanted to take a year off to travel and get a break from the routine of studying before embarking on the six-year program. She asked that her place in the entering class and the financial aid that had been promised be held until the next year. The registrar spoke to Ms. Sabin on the telephone and explained that neither place nor funds could be carried over to another year but that she could reapply for admission the following year. The applicant offered to let the registrar know her plans within the next few weeks. Because it was late in the summer and there were students on a waiting list, it was not possible to grant a long delay. She was told that it would be necessary for her to make a decision within two days. She asked whether she could get funds if she waited a year and learned that she would receive funds for the coming school year but no promise could be made for funds for a first year of study in the future. Two days later the applicant called to say that she needed the money and she would enter the first year class to which she had been accepted. She was asked to send a written statement about her intention to attend school twelve days hence in order to counteract her previously suggested withdrawal. She said that the school could accept her word. The request for a written statement was repeated. She wrote, "I will be there to register on September 4th."

For the entering class, 102 students had been accepted and had confirmed their acceptance. The day for registration arrived. And just before it ended late in the afternoon a count was done of those who had enrolled. There were 99 names on the list. It had been known earlier that one student would be undergoing surgery on the day of matriculation. The name of another student who had held acceptances to more than one school, and had been expected to ask for financial aid but had not done so, was not on the list. The third absentee was Ms. Sabin.

A quick call to another medical school concerning the applicant with multiple acceptances elicited the happy reply from the registrar being called, "Of course _____ has registered here!" But when that registrar learned their new first-year student had made no attempt to notify or withdraw from the school that was calling, she sizzled. It is not surprising that the people at the school that had been jilted were relieved not to have in their class a person with so little regard for the feelings of others, especially students who had not been lucky enough to get an acceptance and were on a waiting list. An excellent replacement for the errant physician-to-be was obtained immediately.

What about Ms. Sabin? She arrived—the last of the entering class to enroll. Her car had broken down.

13. Long-haired Bertram Laennec, neatly combed, tieless, wearing a well-kempt battle jacket over an open-necked khaki shirt tucked into clean jeans that descend to leather boots, is a no-pretense applicant from a state school. His common sense and honesty make up for his lack of verbal polish. The 21-year-old son of a factory foreman and a mother who holds a clerical job is the first, and probably the only one, of three siblings to go to college. He knows from his father's and his own firsthand experience what it is like to work at a boring job. Because he needed money he worked summers after high school and during college as a stock boy in a department store, a bus boy in a restaurant, and a factory hand in a company that made organs. In addition he did lawn maintenance all four years. The work in the factory was dull. He observed that, in general, very few people do the work they want to do, maybe only five or ten percent. His father is luckier than most men in the organ factory — he can avoid the assembly line because he has the skill to do the wiring required for coordination of the pipes and therefore can put the parts of the organ together into a console instead of carrying out a tedious, one-step job.

Young Mr. Laennec was interested in science and had enrolled initially in a technical institute in a large city. In his two years there he earned a straight A average studying biology, chemistry, physics, mathematics, history, western civilization, and German. Because of the absence of social contacts, especially the opportunity to meet girls, he transferred to a public university near his home. He had been pleased to find an expanded curriculum and continued his good scholastic record while studying social science, additional courses in chemistry, and electrical engineering. His grade point average was 3.9; his percentile scores on the MCAT were verbal 90, quantitative 85, general information 97, and science 99. He had been invited to join an honorary scholastic society but declined for two reasons: the fee was $18 and he did not believe in self-congratulatory societies.

While in college Mr. Laennec made regular visits to an adjacent town in which many disadvantaged families lived. There he tutored a seventh grader who objected to the rigidity of his school. The tutor put together a crystal set and gave it to the child to take apart and then helped him put it together. Mr. Laennec swam competitively at the first college he had attended but pointed out that he had been on the team not because he was a great swimmer but because the school needed an additional body in the long distance events. He plays the piano and the trumpet — not well enough to be a professional musician, he says — and is a member of the college band and of an orchestra that accompanies musical productions at the YMCA. He got his interest in music from his father who plays the bass fiddle. Once he traveled to the West Indies to visit a friend. He bicycled, learned folk dancing, and joined a singles club. The latter step was an important one because it enabled him for the first time in his life to have a serious man-woman relationship that he mentioned in another context while discussing caring for people, being a physician, and furthering human happiness.

Mr. Laennec has not done any laboratory research nor worked in a hospital. He is determined to become a physician, probably an ophthalmologist, because of his empathy for the blind. He is especially interested in devices that employ tactile stimuli in combination with a television setup for transferring signals to the brain to help the blind to "see." He wants to go to a medical school that has a good department of ophthalmology because he believes it is necessary to get postgraduate clinical training at the same institution at which one has studied for the medical degree. That naive belief might be a result of his not having had any association with a medical school or a hospital. His recommendations were excellent and he was considered the best premedical applicant from his university.

Mr. Laennec was evaluated by three people because the first two interviewers held widely divergent opinions. One thought he was a little unusual but would be a conscientious student who might have to work hard but who was determined, sensible, and pleasant. Furthermore, there had not been many applicants from his school. The other interviewer thought he was peculiar. Certainly he was not an impeccably dressed, smoothly articulate candidate. Was there something strange about him? Something out of the ordinary about his affect? He was not out of touch with reality; his smiling was never inappropriate. His seemingly self-deprecatory remarks about not having good racing times in swimming or not being a professional musician indicated straightforwardness and not lack of confidence. But hadn't he written under Medical History of Applicant: "child psychologist at age 10 or so for problem in adjusting to puberty"? Yes he had, but only one interviewer had sought an explanation for that statement. His mother, with a strong religious background, had seen him masturbating and had taken him to a psychologist who explained that it was normal.

The interviewer who had asked the applicant about the consultation with a psychologist had not discussed the man-woman relationship with the applicant. Did the undiscerning interviewer know that the woman in the man-woman relationship had died and that the man had felt no remorse? No.

A third interview was arranged. On the appointed day, five minutes after the scheduled hour, a fresh interviewer opened his door to find a young man hunkered down on his heels who rose and spoke in a surly manner about having been kept waiting. Later the interviewer reported that the applicant was indeed strange. He was rejected.

14. Althea Dimas, bright, interesting, and 21, won a Fulbright Scholarship to attend college in the United States after taking third place among 2,000 participants in a nationwide mathematical competition in her country of origin. She had lived for three years under a dictatorship and, after coming to the United States, had applied to become a citizen, as has her 25-year-old brother, a graduate student in physics with whom she shares an apartment in order to cut down expenses. Brother and sister are planning to bring their father and mother to this country to live.

Ms. Dimas is majoring in biology and has earned a grade point average of 3.8. During her first two years in college, in addition to studying, she wrote and directed a play entitled *Coup d' Etat*, inspired by the music of Theodorakis. She knows Greek, Latin, Italian, and German in addition to English and earns money giving private lessons in English to citizens of her native country when she returns home in the summer. She has worked as a volunteer in a hospital in the city where her parents live. During the school year, between classes, she drops in at a nearby hospital in a disadvantaged area near the university to work as a volunteer a few times each week.

She has been on the dean's list, is a member of a national honorary biological society, has served as vice-president of an international relations club that provides opportunities for foreign students to get together for dinner and talks, and has been on a women's student council that discusses the problems of female students on campus. She is happy to be attending college in this country and not living under a dictatorship. At the university, people have been helpful. Some have taught her how to use a microtome, prepare sections of tissue for electron microscopy, and develop the resulting pictures. She seems to be learning new things all the time. She has obtained A's in most of her subjects, including foreign languages, philosophy, social sciences, art, and the premedical courses of chemistry, physics, and mathematics. She is a paid tutor in calculus. Money is a big problem for her. All of her college education has been paid for by American scholarships and the income she earns from small jobs, such as tutoring and working in the college library. She criticizes the lack of health care in the big city in which she lives. She has had to apply for welfare and is receiving Medicaid because she cannot afford the state school's charge for comprehensive health care.

Ms. Dimas has wanted to become a physician since childhood, is especially interested in the social and societal aspects of medicine, and thinks she might want to get a master's degree in public health together with the medical degree. What she wants to do most is to become a physician and to take part in politics. She was an admirer of Dr. Salvador Allende Gossens and of Indira Gandhi and hopes somehow to combine her interests in politics with medicine; for example, in community health care, especially in an urban center where she could work in a city hospital.

Ms. Dimas has entered the interviewer's office carrying a copy of the *New York Times*. She said that she has to keep up with current events, and it is clear that starting the day with the front page and editorial page is a necessity for her. This candidate is bright, interesting, thoughtful, talented; talking with her is fun. Her skill in English runs a close second to that in her native tongue.

At a decision-making meeting of the admissions committee she was marked for acceptance. A question was asked about the percentile rating in the MCAT: verbal 05, quantitative 16, general information 53, and science 78. In answer to the question, one interviewer said he had read the scores and thought they were not significant in the case of an individual who had come from a non-English-speaking country and obtained almost a 4.0 average in college. Another interviewer had simply forgotten about the MCAT while focusing on the candidate's excellent work in college, personal qualifications, and demonstration of talent in writing and directing a musical production. The consensus was that the unsatisfactory performance on the MCAT was not acceptable. A decision was made to ask the applicant to repeat the examination and a letter was sent requesting that she take the test the next time it was given. The answer? There was none. Ms. Dimas enrolled in another medical school.

15. Bruce Simpson, a wide-awake young man of 20 with an unmistakable southern accent, has the build of an athlete and the ambition of a scholar. He was named for a physician who had taught his physician-father and there is no doubt that medicine is a goal of long standing. He will be graduated from college after three years of study, including summer sessions for two years, with a Bachelor of Arts degree in biology and a 4.0 average. His A's were collected in the regular premedical courses of chemistry, physics, calculus, and, of course, his major interest, biology, as well as in many subjects encompassing the humanities and the social sciences. He had not emphasized the hard sciences.

His percentile scores on the MCAT—verbal 85, quantitative 78, general information 74, and science 96—were not as spectacular as his grades but were good. In his last semester at college he planned to do a project in botany in which an attempt would be made to localize a photosensitive substance that was probably involved in the membranous structure of algae.

The applicant's extracurricular activities included tutoring elementary school children during his second year of college, serving as a volunteer in a university hospital during one summer while attending school, working at road construction another summer, and playing intramural basketball and football for one year. He worked as a laboratory instructor in biology and is a member of an honor society. One of his most interesting accomplishments is being a magician. Although he considers himself an amateur, he is not only versed in the lore of that profession but is also a performer. He excelled in athletics in high school and is determined to excel in medicine.

Mr. Simpson's desire is not to be a private practitioner but to be an academician, a worthwhile teacher and clinical investigator, at a university hospital. Clinical research would reinforce his ability to teach. His immediate aim is to be admitted to a good medical school—he already has been accepted by several—and later to take graduate training at a good teaching hospital to attain his ultimate goal. He has thought a lot about his career and the best way to implement it. The recommendations from his professors of chemistry, mathematics, history, and other subjects are splendid.

Mr. Simpson was put on the waiting list but eventually enrolled in another school.

16. Elizabeth Lewis is 23, a graduate of a coeducational university in the East and an attractive person from the standpoints of appearance, verbal expression, and motivation. She is determined to become a physician. What would she do if she were not accepted into medical school? She immediately answered that she would study for another year and reapply. She also pointed out that such a course would not be necessary because she already has been accepted into a medical school but, in her opinion, not as good as that at which she is being interviewed.

Her interest in medicine is not long standing. Early in college she had thought about majoring in biology but switched to anthropology after inauspicious results in a course in biological science. Her grade point average was between 3.3 and 3.4 and her percentile scores on the MCAT were verbal 99, quantitative 85, general information 87, and science 86. While an undergraduate she had earned mostly B's and B+'s except for A's in half of her large number of courses in anthropology and those in art history.

Her father is a professor of history; her mother, considered intelligent and capable by the daughter, is at the age at which some women feel that it is a mistake not to develop a career independent of marriage. The family—father, mother, and siblings—has a strong tradition of involvement in the humanities. Ms. Lewis obtained some familiarity about medicine from a brother-in-law who is a physician.

In college Ms. Lewis took part in a community service organization, served on the student union committee, helped at a draft information service, and worked in the election campaigns of 1968 and 1972. She had also been a counselor at camp. In the summer following her sophomore year she went on an archeological dig in Greece. The latter experience gave her the opportunity to decide whether or not she wanted to be an archeologist. The summer had been interesting, she had learned a lot, and she had decided not to become an archeologist; she could not rationalize spending her life in a career that would be primarily of benefit to herself when so many people lived in unsatisfactory conditions. She thought about going to graduate school or about joining the Peace Corps or Vista. Medicine did not enter her mind until her senior year. At that time she decided to take courses in math and science immediately after obtaining the Bachelor of Arts degree. She had made up her mind to enter the field of medicine.

During the summer after graduation and again in the following year she attended a school recognized for its good summer program. There she completed the science requirements for premedical students with A's in physics, mathematics, and one biology course and B's in another course in biology and in chemistry. In addition she devoted a considerable amount of time to working in hospitals in a preceptor program and helping in an emergency room over a period of 18 months.

Ms. Lewis is bright, goodlooking, and pleasant; she will be a knowledgeable and likable physician. Her scores on the MCAT are fine and her grades are reasonable.

One of the people who interviewed her was an epidemiologist whose knowledge of archeology was as precise as that concerning the spread of disease. He asked the applicant about the findings that were made during the digs in Greece and their location in time. She described the discovery of pieces of pottery and gave a date for their origin that placed the shards within the Stone Age. But when she described the period as Mycenaean, the time of the Greek Heroic age, the interviewer recognized that her knowledge was faulty. The artifacts found on the dig were most likely from a much later period. Could she have meant the Iron Age? Ms. Lewis could not explain the significance of the material, nor was there evidence to indicate that she had read or studied the subject. The inescapable conclusion: she was a dilettante just doing something for diversion during a summer. The interviewer would not support the candidate and she was given a low rating on the waiting list.

Ms. Lewis had a lot of attributes and was admitted to another medical school.

17. Paul Redi comes across as an alert, forceful young man of 21 who is enrolled at a Catholic university. He is direct, unafraid to talk but not verbose. Unlike most preprofessional students he has logged at least as many credit hours in a second subject of interest, chemistry, as he has gained in his major field of biology. Other courses indicate a wide interest in the humanities. His grade point average in science was 3.6 and his cumulative average was 3.7 with the following percentile rating on the MCAT: verbal 99, quantitative 89, general information 94, and science 99.

The applicant has already been accepted at a medical school in his home state, but he declares a strong preference to attend the school that he is visiting for two reasons. One he belittles as being crass: he would be eligible for a name scholarship funded by a former alumnus who had lived in the same county as he had. Residence in that county is one requirement for eligibility for the scholarship; another requirement is that the applicant be a male. The second reason, but one must not assume that it is second in importance, is not that the school has a prestigious reputation but that it offers a nonrigid program, small classes, and the opportunity to do research. Although he has not done much research, he wants to become involved in it.

At college Mr. Redi has worked with a member of the faculty on a project that included a review of the literature on human population growth and an analysis of the growth of beetles on manure. The advisor had become persona non grata at the college because of his outspoken remarks about zero population growth and pollution. Another project was carried out in the clinical laboratories of a hospital in which the applicant calibrated a spectroscopic apparatus in order to measure lead and other heavy ions in human blood. Although his chief interest is to deliver health care in some kind of group practice, he wants to be exposed to research while at medical school because his plans for the future are open.

Mr. Redi has worked during the summers as a technician in a photography laboratory, an assembler in a factory, and a construction worker. Did he get anything out of those jobs in addition to the wages he earned? He learned that the older men worked to support their families and themselves while the younger men could talk about nothing except cars, beer, and sex—and they worked to acquire those ends.

The applicant plays down extracurricular activities at

college—although his list is not small—preferring to avoid "brand names." He believes that students build them up on their applications because they think that is what the medical schools want. He believes that such activities could not be strong if one were taking difficult academic courses. His observations are wise and pungent.

Mr. Redi is cynical but not in the gloomy sense of that word. He is bright and he is aggressive in a productive way. Another interviewer thought the applicant was abrasive and could not second his acceptance. The applicant was snatched by another school and encouraged to enter their Medical Scientist Training Program.

18. Helena Westwood is a blue-eyed, light-haired applicant of 21 years who majored in biology at a college for women noted for turning out leaders. She is wise, pleasant, tactful, and ostensibly calm and self-controlled. The interviewer was obliged to keep her waiting for about ten minutes in order to jot down notes on a preceding applicant. During that hiatus, Ms. Westwood, who was asked to wait in a nearby solarium for patients and relatives, became acquainted with a man receiving experimental therapy for hepatic cancer. Her interest in the patient led to a discussion of clinical research, a subject in which she has not had any experience but in which she is interested.

She is familiar with medical care because her father is a specialist in internal medicine. She describes him as working hard, putting in long hours, taking good care of his patients. She noted with perception that he finds a certain amount of tedium in full-time practice. She herself is strongly motivated to a career in medicine but believes it will be important for her to do research in addition to caring for patients. She knows that her background in science has not been strong, certainly not for involvement in independent research. Except for 32 credit hours in biology, her preparation in science included only the minimal number of subjects required for entrance to medical school; one course had been taken in a low-powered summer session.

After her junior year Ms. Westwood worked during the summer in a laboratory at a university not far from her college. Radioactive precursors of DNA and RNA were used to study sporulation of a bacterium responsible for food poisoning. Perhaps the most rewarding part of that experience was acquiring techniques that became second nature, discovering her own laboratory temperament, and developing favorably in terms of patience, lack of bias, solving problems, and figuring out what to do next. She was excited about the work and found it aesthetically appealing as well as practically significant.

She says that her interest in medicine is principally in research but she wants to go to medical school rather than work for a PhD because a medical education will give her a wider though perhaps less deep scope of knowledge. If she were not accepted into medical school she would work in biology, but she strongly desires a medical career. Her cumulative grade point average was 3.7 and her science average was 4.0. She was initiated into Phi Beta Kappa in her junior year. Her percentile scores on the MCAT were verbal 70, quantitative 85, general information 94, and science 81. The verbal rating was low although an essay she wrote in her application was lucid and interesting. Her extracurricular activities included serving as business manager for her college's junior show in which her job was to raise money from parents and students and, on Saturday mornings, being a student interviewer for the board of admissions—not to recruit students but to give information about the school. During one summer she worked as a laboratory technician and typist in a physician's office. During the summer in which she attended school she also worked as a counter clerk in the kitchen. Hobbies that are important to her include mountain climbing, sailing, and reading.

Ms. Westwood is a bright lady who projects a sense of self-worth and ability to achieve. She did not smoke during the interview—none of the candidates did—and the room was not cold. Yet, when she and the interviewer parted shaking hands, her icy fingers showed the pallor and blue-red blotches of Raynaud's phenomenon. The applicant was accepted.

19. Eric Crane is a 20-year-old neatly dressed, well-spoken young man whose demeanor and discourse reflect his educational background at a well-known preparatory school and an Ivy League college. He wants to continue his association with top-notch institutions by attending the medical school at which he is being interviewed. His agreeable and pleasant personality, coupled with his need to earn money—his father is dead, and his mother is ill—go a long way toward explaining his success as a salesman of dictionaries for three summers during which his door-to-door approach resulted in making almost $3,000—enough to pay almost all his expenses.

In prep school he had earned letters in football and swimming and in college he continued his interest in athletics by playing on two varsity teams. He received a Bachelor of Arts degree, cum laude, in psychology the previous year and applied to medical school then but was not accepted. His cumulative grade point average was 3.1 and in science was 3.0. His first try at the MCAT had been a disaster with percentile scores on the verbal section of 7, quantitative 97, general information 86, and science 24. His premedical advisor hoped that those scores would be essentially disregarded because the applicant had already retaken the test. What had happened was that Mr. Crane took the test on sudden impulse, giving up his place in an important varsity event. He did not even hear the initial instructions and, by misunderstanding, did only one portion of the verbal and did something else incorrectly in the section on science. The scores on the test five months later were verbal 94, quantitative 95, general information 83, and science 94. His academic record showed more passes and high passes than honors and A's.

Between his sophomore and junior years he took a leave of absence and worked as a teacher of mathematics and director of a United States funded agricultural project in an economically and educationally deprived area in a foreign country. In college he served as a volunteer at a mental health center and on the psychiatric ward of a hospital and had been employed as a teacher at a school for disturbed children. He had not been exposed to scientific research, but he had done a study concerned with death, dying, and the treatment of the terminally ill.

Mr. Crane can see himself practicing medicine in another country for awhile or being a psychiatrist or a general practitioner in a rural area. A grandfather had been a physician; an aunt, also a physician, had been on the faculty of a medical school. The applicant particularly liked the intellectual climate of the medical school that he was visiting. He is bright but not brilliant and there is no doubt that he will be a responsible, compassionate, and helpful physician.

Mr. Crane was accepted by at least two other medical schools and he enrolled at a fine one in another part of the country.

20. Mary Lou Cori is a neatly groomed, not very big 21-year-old with zip and sparkle. She is majoring in chemistry and biology at a small college in New England, the same one from which her teacher of biology in high school had been graduated. Her intention is to combine medical research with clinical care, and to achieve this goal she wants to attend a medical school with a strong MD-PhD program. Unlike most applicants to medical school, her interest in research is unusually strong. That interest began during her junior year in high school when she received a grant from the National Science Foundation to study photosynthesis and respiration under the aegis of a pollution control center in another part of the country. She continued her work in air and water pollution for two additional summers. During her sophomore year in college her interests changed to biochemistry. She spent the summer at another college working on enzymes. There she met several premedical and medical students. The summer following her junior year she received a stipend to work at an outstanding biochemical laboratory where she studied DNA replication.

Ms. Cori recognizes that there might be some weakness in her background for investigative work because of the limited facilities at her college. However, she enjoys the relationships formed in the closely knit community and uses her summer vacations to strengthen her preparation for medical and graduate school. The summers have been learning experiences that enforced her determination to have a career that combines biological and biochemical research with solutions to medical problems. She believes that a discovery might be of interest to only a handful of people involved in the project, but of more significance is the possibility of working on something that might benefit many people. She feels that maximum rewards are to be gained in medical research.

Ms. Cori's percentile scores on the MCAT were verbal 51, quantitative 70, general information 43, and science 95. She considered the section on math "dinky" and the science "simple." Although her score on the verbal section was low, two essays included in her application—one to the medical school and the other to the graduate school—were lucid, well-organized, and interesting. Both her cumulative and science grade point averages were 3.9.

Ms. Cori is the president of the chemical society at her college, a member of the physics society and the women's council, a dormitory proctor, a tutor, and an assistant in a laboratory and in a library. Her strong interest in science and her small stature do not keep her from being involved in athletics. She is a member of the varsity field hockey team and the rifle club and plays football and volleyball.

What does she consider her assets? Ms. Cori replied immediately, "I am strongly motivated, don't give up, don't let things get me down. And whatever I do, I try to do to the best of my ability."

Ms. Cori is an intelligent, cheerful, self-assured, highly qualified young woman who could not be content with a career as a general practitioner. She needs the challenge of combining medicine with research. She was accepted by both the medical and the graduate schools, although the acceptance by the graduate school had been slow. Ms. Cori enrolled as a graduate student at a university known for outstanding work in biochemistry. Whether her rejection of the acceptance into the MD-PhD program was based on a stronger desire to do research than to combine research with clinical work, whether it was a result of greater financial support from the other school, or whether it reflected a wish to be in the city in which a close friend worked was not known.

21. Arthur Holmes, age 21, the only child of a salesman and a housewife who did not go to college, is attending an Ivy League school from which he will be graduated at the end of four years with a Bachelor of Arts and Master of Arts degree in the history of science. He is friendly and enthusiastic and declares that nothing gives him more pleasure than helping people, and no career other than medicine offers the opportunity to help others directly while also providing a challenge to intellectual fulfillment.

His cumulative grade point average was 3.7 and his science average of 3.5 included a C+ in organic chemistry. Most of his courses had been in the social sciences and the humanities with few in the physical and biological sciences or mathematics. His scores on the MCAT were in the 90th percentile: verbal 99, quantitative 92, general information 91, and science 93.

Mr. Holmes did research at a cancer institute during two summers, worked as a counselor at a state school for retarded children and as a volunteer in an infirmary, helped in screening for lead poisoning, and taught at a religious school. He played the violin informally and operated a ham radio station.

The applicant's letters of recommendation were laudatory, and one was a profuse exaggeration that characterized the student's research as representing the essentials of a thesis for a PhD. His performance in organic chemistry was attributed to difficulty in taking "a certain kind of quantitative examination" rather than reflecting a lack of knowledge. An instructor wrote that a C+ in organic chemistry from their school was as good as an A from other schools. An outstanding letter came from a professor who had been an ambassador to another country.

Mr. Holmes's goal is clinical practice in a group, not on a fee-for-service basis—perhaps in a health maintenance organization with regular hours. He wants time available to teach at a university and to write on medical topics, especially history and ethics. His honors thesis is going to be on the drug laws of one state.

It is unlikely, on the basis of the interview, that Mr. Holmes will do laboratory research. The subjects he has studied and his personality do not indicate an interest in scientific investigation, but he does seem to be an individual with a strong feeling for people—someone who will be a good physician.

The applicant was accepted by the school at which he was interviewed, as well as by some others, but decided to take a year off to study the humanities abroad. After his return he enrolled at another school.

22. Anna Lyons turned 20 just two months before her interview. She has completed all the requirements for a Bachelor of Arts degree with a triple major—chemistry, zoology, and English—after two years of study at a fine southern university. She has college credit covering 40 courses, 12 of them representing work done at a private secondary school that awarded her advanced placement credit. Three courses had been taken at a small college during the summer before graduation from the secondary school and 7 had been taken during the summers while at the university from which she will receive her degree. Her cumulative grade point average was 3.6 and her average in science was 3.5. Her percentile scores on the MCAT were verbal 88, quantitative 85, general information 97, and science 98. She is applying to the Medical Scientist Training Program in order to get a medical degree and also a PhD degree in pharmacology.

At present Ms. Lyons is enrolled in a graduate school studying several aspects of neuroscience: anatomy, biology, and endocrinology. She has stopped taking courses in English because they ruin her writing but she has written short stories and is working on novels. She likes to analyze peoples' dreams and believes that her interest in the effect of drugs on behavior might lead her into pharmacology and phsychology or psychiatry. She is interested in psychoanalysis and thinks she might want to be a psychiatrist.

Ms. Lyons is wide awake, poised, relaxed, and obviously bright, but it is not easy to get answers from her that are specific. For example, her goal is to teach, do research, and practice medicine—but not all at the same time. That statement seems reasonable enough, but how does she see herself combining those interests? "It would depend on circumstances." She cannot suggest a realistic approach.

The applicant knows that she "likes medicine": she reads articles in a well-known textbook of internal medicine, a cousin is a physician, her father is a pharmacist, and her mother, being intellectually curious, always looks up the family's medical problems in a book. She commented that she had met graduate students in basic sciences who were more excited about things such as recent publications than were medical students who talked about subjects that were not related to medicine and seemed to want to be doing other things.

Her extracurricular activities include working as a laboratory assistant, being a receptionist at a desk in a dormitory, and contributing editorials to the school newspaper published weekly during the summer.

Ms. Lyons gets outstanding marks for intelligence but not for maturity. She is not easy to talk with because she seems cold and remote. In one letter of recommendation she is described as easy to know and to like. The two people who interviewed her, however, agreed with each other and with comments in the candidate's other recommendations noting her intelligence, lack of maturity, and seeming inability to interact with people. Ms. Lyons was accepted by another medical school.

23. Charles Harvey is a 19-year-old senior from an eastern university who will be getting his Bachelor of Arts degree in chemistry at the end of three years of study. He has taken more than the ordinary number of courses each semester and his performance with a heavy load has earned him a cumulative grade point average over 3.6 and a science average over 3.7. All his scores on the MCAT were in the 90th percentile with the quantitative section 98 and the science 99. His recommendations are outstanding and emphasize his intelligence, zeal, and confidence or aggressiveness.

In the interview Mr. Harvey is forceful, vigorous, and determined. He wants, more than anything else in the world, to become a doctor. His interest in mathematics and the sciences is of long standing, and in high school he won a National Science Foundation Scholarship and studied physiological responses of amphibia. Mr. Harvey is not shy about his accomplishments. He wants to be, and considers himself, well rounded. He believes that a physician should know more than just medical subjects and has studied art, literature, music, economics, psychology, sociology, and other topics. He has relatives in the health professions and comments wisely about people's abilities, ambitions, and attainments as well as the role of necessity in thwarting one's goals. He describes, for example, a grandfather—a professional engineer—who, because of the depression in the 1930s took a job with the city in order to support his family. But the grandfather was never satisfied. He was a brilliant man and should have been working with his inventions.

Mr. Harvey is busy apart from his school work. He has served voluntarily as a technician in a bacteriology and serology laboratory, works one afternoon a week as a teaching assistant in a laboratory, is an assistant instructor for beginning swimmers in his college, and has taught swimming at a summer camp. As an Eagle Scout, he works one night every other week with a boy scout troup and during the alternate weeks plays the trumpet in the American Legion Band.

Mr. Harvey is interested in the practice of medicine with the choice of specialty wide open but "probably not psychiatry." He is determined to have a career in clinical medicine but recognizes that he has not been exposed to investigative work and thinks he might be interested in research. He insists that most people go into medicine because they are interested in the subject and not in the financial rewards. He himself comes across strongly as a bright, altruistic, hardworking candidate and competitor. He already has been accepted by two medical schools in a large city but wants to go to the school at which he is being interviewed because he believes that this school and one other get the smartest students and provide the best intellectual atmosphere.

It is clear that Mr. Harvey, with his innate ability and eagerness, will be a hardworking, up-to-date physician who will provide excellent guidance and care for his patients. He was marked for acceptance. Because of the large number of applicants given an *accept* rating at the same time, he became a name on a waiting list that was not tapped. Mr. Harvey enrolled at a school noted for excellence—but not his first choice.

24. Lynn Guthrie, 20 years old, a smiling, bright girl with top-notch grades, has a strong interest in the practical application of medical knowledge. Enrolled at an eastern university, where she will earn a Bachelor of Science degree in chemistry after three years of study, she has achieved a cumulative grade point average of 3.9 and a science average of 4.0. Her percentile scores on the MCAT were verbal 92, quantitative 83, general information 87, and science 91. Ms. Guthrie's excellent performance in science should not be interpreted as indicating an interest in research. Although she worked on a laboratory project in organic chemistry, her goal is to help people through medical care.

The applicant's recommendations are outstanding and her extracurricular activities include tutoring high school students; serving as a representative in dormitory government; working as a laboratory assistant; taking part in dramatic, premedical, and cultural clubs; and sailing.

Ms. Guthrie is easy to talk with and pleasant. She believes firmly in the concept of "man can do." Her altruism extends to man's doing anything and everything. For example, because there is so much to see and do in the world, and so many people to meet, no one should have to sacrifice one minute of his life to a crippling illness. Most people are born with the opportunity to live life as fully and as rigorously as they choose. Man can become a teacher, an artist, or a physician, and in the latter role he can help the physically handicapped to develop all their faculties and go out into the world to discover what is waiting to be seen and appreciated. Man as teacher and physician can move mountains. The applicant's belief in the power of education and healing to solve society's problems is not a new one. In this beautiful scheme there is no place for economic necessity or inherent difference in ability. Another assumption in her theory of life is equality at birth. All individuals, for example, children from age four, if given direction, can accomplish much. The interviewer suggests going back to two years of age or even day one to allow for early nuturing in order to help her theory of equality at birth. The applicant believes that if people are given educational and medical help they will be able to discover the good things in the world. Monetary considerations do not play a role. As an offshoot of this discussion, the interviewer asks the applicant how many people in this country does she think are satisfied with their jobs? Ms. Guthrie answers that four-fifths of the people are not just satisfied but actually like their jobs.

The interviewer recognizes and worries when personal bias comes into play. Sometimes the interviewer allows prejudice to poke a hole: would the applicant consider using the impersonal pronoun *one* occasionally instead of referring to *man* doing this and *man* doing that? "No" was the answer. She does not like using *one* in speech or in writing.

The applicant is not simply enthusiastic and naive but perhaps lacking in experience and depth of judgment. It is clear that she can handle an academic program with ease and that she likes developing relationships with people. She is a good candidate and there is no doubt that she will be accepted into a medical school. Her innate intelligence, ability to work hard, and friendliness are fine qualities. Perhaps wisdom must wait for development of maturity. Until then, she is staking all on man as physician solving the problems of the sick, the handicapped, our society, and the world.

Ms. Guthrie enrolled in the medical school of the university where she was completing her premedical studies.

25. Stanley Bernard, a friendly young man of 20, arrives casually at the interviewer's office. He is a little late, probably as a result of the interviewer's not getting straight the time schedule for the interview. His special interest in medicine is clinical practice as a family doctor in a small town. He does not know if that practice will include surgery. Another thought he is holding about medicine is to become the director of the United States Public Health Service. It occurs to the interviewer that he just might make it because he is a hard worker and because of his particular interest. Indeed, he wants to attend a medical school in proximity to a school of public health, and he wants to be the very best doctor and public health servant possible. Another wish is that the medical school be near a large city that he and his wife-to-be can visit and enjoy cultural events such as the theatre.

His plans for the future include marrying a woman older than he is who will teach in high school while he attends medical school. She will support him and herself while he pursues his medical studies. Then, when Mr. Bernard serves his internship, he will be earning $8,000, enough for him and his wife, who will be close to 30 years of age, to begin a family.

Mr. Bernard expects to receive a Bachelor of Science degree in biology and already has been elected to Phi Beta Kappa. His grade point average in science was 4.0 and his cumulative average was 3.8. He has studied the required premedical subjects plus courses in psychology, sociology, politics, logic, literature, music, religion, philosophy, and art history. His program of study could be considered average for premedical students from the standpoint of the types and degree of difficulty of courses taken during a four year period. His performance is above average but does not reflect unique ability. His percentile scores on the MCAT were verbal 61, quantitative 82, general information 87, and science 86. He has taken part in a research project in water pollution and analyzed samples of water; he also has been involved in collecting data on the numbers of hospitals, beds, and physicians in the city where his college is located.

Extracurricular activities included membership on an ecology committee, a socio-religious group, a house council, and honorary societies. As a member of a marching band and a concert band, he played the saxophone and oboe and had played the organ as an accompanist for a musical production at his college. He was the treasurer of a fraternity and an alternate on an advisory committee to a bookstore. He was the advertising manager for the student newspaper and had been an instructor in three laboratories at college. During the summers he had worked in a pharmacy and also in a hospital as an orderly on a floor and in an emergency room. The most interesting, and shocking, thing he had ever done was to attend autopsies.

The applicant is strongly motivated for a career in medicine and does not have to consider an alternative goal because he already has been accepted by three medical schools but wants most to attend the school at which he is being interviewed. In his recommendations his persistence and perserverance as well as his intelligence were de-scribed. He is well qualified and has shown himself to be a hard worker and a good student. He is not different from other good students. In one enthusiastic recommendation a minor shortcoming was mentioned; namely, that Mr. Bernard continually chattered about everything and anything but that he would outgrow this propensity as he matured. That gift of the gab was much in evidence throughout the interview. He was smart enough and eager enough—but oh, if only he didn't talk so much!

Mr. Bernard enrolled at another school.

26. Joan Hardy, a 21-year-old student who had been first in her class of 465 at a high school in the Midwest, is majoring in biochemistry at a college for women in the East. She is well groomed and her straight blond hair hangs neatly over her shoulders. It is easy to talk with Ms. Hardy as she projects an air of self-confidence, capability, and resourcefulness. Her father is an engineer, her mother an assistant principal in a high school—and Ms. Hardy is used to achieving. She began the study of a musical instrument in second grade and plays the organ in a church. She is a member of the crew on her college's team, served as vice-president in a college house, and is a teaching assistant in a science laboratory.

Ms. Hardy has one sibling, a brother who is studying medicine at another school. Her own interest in medicine evolved through her study of biology in high school. Now, in her last year of college, she is working on an honors project in biochemistry; if she could have one wish fulfilled, it would be to devote all her time to completing that work without distractions. Her determination as shown in her desire to finish the project seems likely to carry through in a medical career. Her major interest in medicine, however, is not research but clinical practice, possibly in a hospital setting.

Ms. Hardy's percentile scores on the MCAT were verbal 83, quantitative 74, general information 57, and science 89. Her science grade point average was 3.6 and her cumulative average was 3.5. Ms. Hardy was asked her opinion about the MCAT. She answered, ''If it's a good day, one does great.'' She thinks that the verbal section is not as extensive as that in the Scholastic Aptitude Test; that the math is strictly at the level of that studied in high school with no calculus or trigonometry; that the section on science requires knowledge of college biology, chemistry, and physics; and that to do well in the part on general information one would "need a course in everything!"

Ms. Hardy was accepted.

27. Harold Frank had been number one in his class of 90 students—45 males and 45 females—at a preparatory school; now he is attending a prestigious unversity. He is a pleasant 22-year-old with a good but not outstanding academic average. Although his cumulative grade point average at college was 3.6 and his science average 3.2, his grades had fallen progressively from his first year through his third. He is pursuing a major in social relations and has taken 14 courses in social studies; two in chemistry; and one each in biology, physics, expository writing, English, and Hebrew. His scores on the MCAT were in the 90th percentile except for a 74 in science.

Mr. Frank's interest in medicine surfaced after his sophomore year. Before then he had planned to prepare himself for a career in clinical psychology. During the summer following his second year in college, he took part in a program at a state hospital for patients with psychiatric problems. He lived at the hospital, worked on a ward, and had the opportunity to attend classes and discussions with members of the staff. The emphasis was on modification of behavior. Conversations with psychologists and psychiatrists, in addition to reading, convinced him that the image of the physician was better than that of the psychologist. As a practicing physician he could do more to help people with emotional problems than he could by offering talking cures as a psychologist. He decided to identify with the role of the psychiatrist. His stated goal is to be engaged in the clinical practice of psychiatry, perhaps combined with research. What he means by research is not clear.

During the time that Mr. Frank was preparing for college, he worked hard for an organization interested in raising money for a religious cause. In his freshman year at college he served as a consultant to a similar group on the campus—no leg work involved. In his sophomore year he worked one afternoon a week at a day-care center and in his junior year he tutored a child at a school for the retarded.

The applicant has not applied to the excellent medical school at the university at which he is doing his undergraduate work because his first choice is the school that he is visiting. The interviewer wondered silently whether that was the real reason or whether the candidate recognized that his university might not look with favor upon his application in view of his downhill performance.

What does he know about the school at which he is being interviewed? Nothing specific. Yet he knows that he will be happiest in the environment here? Yes—because "those things filter down." He can't put "it" or "those things" into words. Another topic: has he ever worked on a project completely on his own, at any stage of his life? Yes—he read all the *OZ* books as a child.

One interviewer was strongly supportive of the applicant. The other interviewer thought the candidate was a sweet guy who was qualified to study medicine but was not in the same league as were other applicants. Because of the divergence of opinions and the insistence of one member of the admissions committee, another interview was given. The third interviewer thought the applicant was wonderful to talk to and a highly creative man. So the applicant was accepted.

28. Rose Mahoney has been interested in medicine since childhood but had not seriously considered entering that profession because her parents did not plan on her going to college. The family background is a modest one in which even a high school education is a rarity. Money was saved for a son to attend college but not for the older daughter. The son, who did not want to study, was encouraged by the parents to go to college. He entered, dropped out, and became a golf pro. The daughter, after being graduated from high school at the age of 17, decided to pursue a career in nursing. She took the academic route and earned a Bachelor of Science degree in nursing after four years of study at a state university. She became actively engaged in professional nursing as a staff nurse at a busy hospital in a large city and also as a nurse-teacher. While holding responsible positions, her goals and expectations changed. As a mature adult, she wanted a role in which she could use her initiative and exert independent action: she wanted to be a physician.

Ms. Mahoney, however, was married to a medical student and her salary was their sole source of income. In addition to that consideration, funds would be needed for her to return to college and study the courses required for entrance to medical school. Because of the stringent financial situation, the goal of becoming a physician had to be abandoned. An opportunity for graduate study in nursing, with full tuition and a stipend, was offered. She took that alternative and obtained a Master of Science degree in medical and surgical nursing. During the following two years she was a member of the faculty at a college and at a medical school. After her husband earned his medical degree, and while he was serving his military obligations, Ms. Mahoney enrolled at a state university 60 miles from her husband's post and commuted 120 miles daily in order to complete the premedical science courses.

Ms. Mahoney is an alert, well-groomed young woman of 30 who has the appearance and enthusiasm of a college student. As an undergraduate she had taken part in several extracurricular activities; for example, student government and a committee on international relations. She was treasurer of the student finance committee, president of her sorority and of the student nurses association, chairperson of Parents Weekend and Junior Week, and a member of the dean's committee on improvement of the curriculum. She served voluntarily in a hospital; worked to earn money during the academic year; and in the summers was employed as a waitress, receptionist, nurse's aide, and residence counselor. She had been a member of the National Educational Honor Society and had done library research on communicable diseases that resulted in development of a policy manual on the control of infections.

Ms. Mahoney's motivation for a medical career is strong. She feels that her past education and experiences would serve her well in the medical profession as a physician. Her cumulative grade point average as an undergraduate was 3.1 and, as a graduate student, 3.8. Her average in science was 2.8 as an undergraduate and 4.0 as a graduate student. Her percentile scores on the MCAT taken eight months before completion of her premedical courses were verbal 71, quantitative 15, general information 67, and science 27. Her interview took place after the class to which she was applying for admission had been accepted. She did not succeed in gaining admission to any medical school. It is likely that her performance in the quantitative and science sections of the MCAT prevented her acceptance.

29. Evan Childs is an attractively garbed youth of 20 who is bright enough on paper to arouse the interest of an admissions committee but not eager or compulsive enough to make an effort to impress two interviewers by arriving on time. One would hope that a candidate from a relatively nearby school would check travel schedules carefully, allowing for the inclemencies of winter and the vagaries of the railroad, and not play the trains so closely as to risk arriving an hour late.

Mr. Childs will earn a Bachelor of Arts degree in history and science after four years of study with specialization, ostensibly, in pure mathematics. In reality he has become dissatisfied with, and has little interest or skill in, mathematics. After his sophomore year he rediscovered biology, which he had always enjoyed. He became convinced to take a careful look at the medical profession through conversations with premedical fellow students, family doctors, and physician-friends. He is still unfocused as to how to make use of the medical training he is seeking—perhaps pathology, pharmacology, or practice. But he knows that he is ready to dedicate himself to the study of medicine, a subject that seems challenging and variegated. He is particularly interested in the interaction between medicine and society, and he feels that his background in several fields—that is, a liberal education—will put him in a better position to be a useful member of the medical profession.

His transcript shows two semesters of biology and four of mathematics; the expected premedical courses in chemistry and physics but without many letter grades; several courses in history of science and in Japanese; and others in sociology, government, music, and the humanities. His grade point average in science was a satisfactory 3.5 and his cumulative average was a more than satisfactory 3.7 with his strength in Japanese and history of science. His percentile scores on the MCAT were verbal 90, quantitative 61, general information 99, and science 84. He took the test a second time because of the low score in mathematics and raised it to the 80th percentile. He is working on a project for his senior thesis, the subject of which is the introduction of western science and medicine into Japan.

Mr. Child's avocation is music, and his recommendations described him as a violist, pianist, and harpsichordist who performed in the college orchestra and a Bach society and had been associated with an FM radio station. He himself says that he does not play music often. He has been a member of a lightweight crew. During the summers while in college he worked as a clerk in an investment company and as a research assistant in a chemical company.

The applicant's recommendations from his college are good. He is considered intelligent and a thorough worker but not one noted for originality. His record is that of a good but not an outstanding student. In the interview he is pleasant, somewhat self-centered but in no way obnoxious. It is clear that he will have no difficulty as a medical student. Mr. Childs was not accepted by the school that he visited on a stormy winter morning but was accepted at an excellent school.

30. Catherine Vornoskov is a vigorously healthy young woman of 20 years who identifies strongly with her religious, cultural, and geographic background in eastern Europe. She is working for a Bachelor of Arts degree in natural science at a first-rate coeducational university in a large city. She also has studied at four universities in Europe and is fluent in at least five languages. Her science grade point average was 3.6, but the cumulative average, that probably will be as good or better than that in science, was not available because the grades for courses studied abroad were yet to be recorded. However, she has no shortage of excellent credentials for work done in biology, chemistry, physics, and languages in this country. Her percentile scores on the MCAT were verbal 83, quantitative 84, general information 59, and science 74. Ms. Vornoskov's parents were born in another country where her father was trained as a lawyer. He is working as a dairyman in the United States. Her mother obtained a college degree in Europe.

The applicant's extracurricular activities include membership on the varsity squad in badminton, being captain of a volleyball team and coach of a swimming team for girl scouts, and serving as vice-president of a cultural group for students. She has studied art at a school outside the university she is attending and she likes to ski.

Ms. Vornoskov is working on an honors project in physics, measuring the characteristics of gases at low temperatures. Although she can see herself doing research in physics or chemistry, she believes that dealing with people is more interesting and wants to practice medicine in a large city, perhaps in a community similar to that of the family's origin in Europe.

The applicant has outstanding recommendations and is bright, eager, and straightforward. In summary, she is a solid candidate who will perform well in medical school and be a most competent physician. She was given a high place on the waiting list but withdrew after being accepted at an excellent medical school.

31. When Timothy Boyle, a 21-year-old student from a small city university in the Midwest, is welcomed to the interview, his hand is wringing wet, yet the interview is not at all strained or tense. Mr. Boyle, who is completing the requirements for a Bachelor of Science degree in biology and natural science at the end of his third year of study, is a pleasant young man who speaks quietly but with conviction. His deep sense of social responsibility to people who need medical care comes through clearly; his goal is to become involved in family practice in the rural areas of Appalachia.

During the three months between graduation from high school and entering the university he had taken part in a program sponsored by the governor of his state in which he served as an intern to the director of the department of natural resources. He traveled widely to represent the department, co-chaired a task force in long-range environmental planning, and reviewed legislation for a member of the state's house of representatives. Other governmental activities included helping to design a nonpartisan system for voter registration in the city in which he attended school and, in the year of a presidential election, serving as the canvass director of a congressional district's presidential campaign. He enjoyed working with as many as fifty people a day, investigating public opinion, and recognized that personal action is capable of solving community problems.

In carrying out a research project in political sciene, Mr. Boyle described a general mathematical model that could be used for voting behavior. In order to predict at a practical level how people would vote, the model would require computer techniques. During two of the summers of his college years he had raised a large garden that was worth $500 and worked fifteen hours a week on the family's farm.

The applicant has been accepted by two medical schools in his home state. One of the reasons that he wants to study medicine at the school at which he is being interviewed is to get away from the conservative political climate of the Midwest and be able to experience the liberal climate of the Northeast. His aim after completion of medical school is to take a two-year internship or do postgraduate work in the region familiar with the medical problems of the people he wants to help.

Mr. Boyle's cumulative and science grade point averages were 3.8. His percentile scores on the MCAT were verbal 88, quantitative 70, general information 93, and science 93. His chief academic interest is evolving into biochemistry and he is meeting the challenge of biosynthesis of some organic compounds. Although his interest in science is strong, his felt need, based on ethical sensibility, is stronger. He is geared to a career in applied medicine in order to help people in disadvantaged areas.

Mr. Boyle, who observed that politics and medicine have one thing in common—"the need to get along with people"—was accepted.

32.   Nora Bron is a cheerful, enthusiastic 22-year-old woman who is majoring in chemistry at an eastern university. Her academic program in science includes more difficult courses than those customarily selected by premedical students. Her cumulative grade point average of 3.17 and her average of 3.0 in science were below the mean of candidates accepted during the previous year at the school to which she is applying. Her percentile scores on the MCAT, however, were excellent with a verbal of 99, quantitative 93, general information 98, and science 91.

Ms. Bron is pleasant and eager to talk about her love of science. As far back as she can remember she has liked science. For example, at the age of three she took apart flowers. She did not tear them apart; she examined them. At the age of four she disassembled and put back together an alarm clock. When six years old she dissected chicken hearts saved by her mother before cooking the family's meal. The first abstract concept that she can recollect is that of parallel lines when, again at the age of six, she drew two lines side by side in the sand and realized that the lines would not meet.

After being graduated from high school she received funding from the National Science Foundation and the American Cancer Society to do independent research that resulted in a publication. The interviewer said that it must have been exciting to see her first publication; but Ms. Bron says that she did not see it, that perhaps it was included in a paper describing the results of multiple investigators sponsored by the American Cancer Society. Another publication is a coloring book promoting good health habits for children. During her junior year at college she worked as a laboratory assistant for a graduate student and did the computer analysis of intramolecular stress on photosynthetically formed diradicals. During her senior year she hopes to finish a book that will serve as a mathematical study aid for a course in quantum mechanics.

Her extracurricular activities include serving as a representative to a student union; being a wardrobe mistress for a college drama society; and working one summer as a cook, tutor, and baby-sitter for three families. She has lined up a position as a volunteer in a day-care center during the next semester.

Ms. Bron says that her passion is people but that science is her love. That is, she wants to bring her scientific knowledge into medicine but does not want to do scientific investigation. Her goal is clinical care, perhaps in pediatrics or pediatric psychiatry. She would like to join a private group that works on a fee-for-service basis. Her parents have civil service jobs and she has had enough experience to be shy about what might happen to patients under government control.

The applicant is highly familiar with the educational system at the school that she is visiting. When she first read the description of the school's program in the catalog, she believed that she had found the answer to what she visualized the ideal medical school to be.

The interview was long and circumlocutious. Some things had not meshed; others had been interesting and probably correct. The applicant was obviously a hard worker and conscientious. The interviewer was not sure how smart she was and wondered what the other interviewer would say about the candidate at the next meeting of the admissions committee. He said very little, but it was a lot. He simply chopped her. She was accepted by a medical school at a good private university.

33. Jon Steinmetz, 21, is easy to talk with, being pleasant, direct, and quick thinking. He majored in electrical engineering at an eastern university and attained a grade point average in science of 3.7 and a cumulative average of 3.67. His percentile scores on the MCAT were 96 in the quantitative and science sections and lower in the verbal and general information. His recommendations are very good.

As Mr. Steinmetz took courses in biology, he began to study models of the human arterial tree. Then, using a previously constructed model, he carried out an independent project that combined his knowledge of electrical engineering with that of human biology. His model represents the cardiovascular system with a generator to simulate the heart and electrical transmission lines to represent the blood vessels. He is able to relate voltage to blood pressure, current to blood flow, and viscosity to resistance and can hook up any part of the circuit and equate it to physiological phenomena. The project seems interesting to the listener, but the plethora of small details required to get the model to work has not been interesting to the student. The network is complex and in trying to simplify it he got bogged down in boring statistics. Mr. Steinmetz is completely honest. He knows that his background in engineering might be useful in medicine, but he is not keen on applying that training to medicine. His goal is clinical practice.

The best part of Mr. Steinmetz's life has been going to college but he has also enjoyed traveling across the country while in high school. He has worked hard in service and construction jobs to earn money during every vacation period while in college. He plays the guitar, is an amateur photographer, and is a member of several honorary fraternities.

The candidate is intelligent, stable, mature, and capable of hard work. His interest in people and in medical practice is high. Because of the crush of applicants, he was put on a waiting list. He attended another school.

34. Ruth Lambert is a 22-year-old soft-spoken, unassuming, highly intelligent young woman. Not given to garrulity, but a deep thinker, she was graduated with highest honors from a small coeducational college in the East where she majored in history with a minor in economics and had grade point averages, both cumulative and in science, of 3.9. Her percentile scores on the MCAT were verbal 99, quantitative 95, general information 97, and science 96. As a postbaccalaureate undergraduate, she is enrolled in premedical courses.

In college Ms. Lambert's scholarly interests precluded active participation in campus life. However, she tutored remedial reading once a week and taught French and German in an Upward Bound program. Later, she worked as a volunteer in an outpatient clinic at a hospital.

Because of Ms. Lambert's skill in writing, evident from the essay in her application, the interviewer asked about experience in journalism. Yes, she had written a historical short story, based upon a biblical figure, that she had not attempted to publish. The story was so esteemed by her advisor in history that it was placed in the college library where it is often read.

What did the applicant find most interesting about going to college? Developing relationships with people. She had been encouraged to follow an academic career but had not considered medicine. Indeed, except for mathematics, she had not taken any courses in college that would fulfill the premedical requirements for science. In the last half of her college career, she met premedical students and talked to some whose parents were doctors. The scholarly options opened to her began to pall and she began to think about medicine—a profession that requires service and provides intellectual challenge and a variegated life. She made the decision to complete her honors program in the humanities and postpone the study of basic sciences until after graduation. Now, at the time of the interview, she is completing her premedical requirements at a university where her husband is a graduate student in biology.

Ms. Lambert does not want to do graduate work or research, but she likes the graduate-type of approach to studying and the de-emphasis on examinations at the school at which she is being interviewed. She is emphatic, in a quiet way, about wanting more than anything else to become a practicing physician. She has already been accepted by two medical schools.

The applicant was accepted by the school that she was visiting. After her acceptance she withdrew to attend another school where her husband plans to continue his work.

35. David Jenner, age 20, is a gracious young man with easy composure who had attained a superior record at a college where it is possible to acquire simultaneously a solid education in the liberal arts and sciences and in religious studies. The latter included analyses of classical texts in their original languages in order to deepen the student's ethical and philosophical values. The combined secular and religious program demanded ten hours of classroom instruction daily. Mr. Jenner earned 3.7 cumulative and science grade point averages with good scores on the MCAT: verbal 97, quantitative 61, general information 91, and science 89. His major in premedicine is strong in biology and includes the expected courses in physics, mathematics, and chemistry plus biochemistry and the humanities.

Mr. Jenner has done laboratory research, testing for antibodies, and also has been a member of a delegation that makes weekly visits to hospitals and orphanages to share kind words and smiles with the unfortunate occupants. He quotes Hippocrates's observation that ''some patients, though conscious that their condition be perilous, recover their health simply through their contentment with their physician.''

The applicant's goal is to be in practice outside a big city but close enough to be able to work at a hospital as a teacher and perhaps as an investigator. He believes that doing research is a good way to keep up to date. A relative is a physician and several of his friends are medical students.

In addition to being a serious student who clearly shows an interest in helping people, he has been a swimming instructor at a summer camp, an advisor to a nature club, and a counselor in religious studies. His recommendations are excellent. He is an attractive person with a strong motivation for medical school and has already been accepted at one school but hopes to enter the school at which he is being interviewed. He is a fine candidate. Because of the number of applicants, he was put on a waiting list. He enrolled at another school.

36. Jane Curie, a lilliputian applicant of 22 years, had been described in one letter as shy. Shy indeed! She is neither bashful nor hesitant nor timid. Little time is required to recognize her as a low-keyed but interesting conversationalist who is friendly and wide awake. A senior student attending a small college in New England, she will receive a Bachelor of Science degree with a joint major in biology and chemistry. Her academic record places her at the top of her class and it is fun to count her grades: ten A+'s, nine A's, three B+'s, two Honors, and a science grade point average of 4.0 and a cumulative average of 3.9 with eight courses in progress. She has studied, in addition to her courses in science, a foreign language, economics, literature, art, and geography. Her percentile scores on the MCAT were verbal 97, quantitative 87, general information 97, and science 99.

Ms. Curie plays the piano and flute and had been a member of her college's football and concert bands during her freshman year. She is a member of a ski team and a mountaineering club and took part in an environmental quality action group. She has been employed regularly in the student dining hall.

During one summer she worked on a research project funded by the National Science Foundation on the effect of nutrition on cancer in animals. Her role was to take care of the rats used in the experiments and perform assays for enzymes. That work on cancer had been exciting enough to make her think seriously about doing research in cancer as well as clinical work in the future. She also had worked on a project at an oceanographic institute, and she described her role accurately as a laboratory technician and not as an independent investigator. In order to achieve her goals of doing clinical work and medical research, she sees herself in the future working in a hospital associated with a medical school.

Ms. Curie's recommendations are first-rate and indicate her intellectual capacities as a college scholar and her ability to work independently. One delightful comment was, "Very simply she is an outstanding student who quietly goes about excelling."

The applicant likes the idea of working on a project, completing it, and writing it up. The requirement of a thesis in medical school does not put her off because she thinks it ties in with the concept of medicine's being a continuing education. She is not a flashy miss but a bright, serious, happy student. She was admitted to the medical school at which she was being interviewed.

37. It is easy to talk with Martin Ross, a pleasant 27-year-old who has been in the schooling business for eleven years since graduation from high school. His activities can be explained in part by the academic degrees collected: a Bachelor of Arts in sociology after four years of study at a fine college and a Master of Arts and a Doctor of Philosophy in sociology after seven years at an outstanding university. During the last two years of his work for the PhD, he completed the required premedical courses.

As an undergraduate, Mr. Ross wrote reviews of books and lectures for the newspaper and literary magazine at his college, acted in plays, and joined a religious-cultural organization. During the summers he had gone to school, been a camp counselor, and done clerical work for a medical group. The theses for his two postgraduate degrees were on the sociology of organizations. Analyzing two large corporations, he compared their goals as money-making businesses and the goals of the individuals who worked for the corporations. In another sociological project he investigated the breakdown of class structure during a time of technological upheaval.

Mr. Ross's grade point average in science was 3.5 and the cumulative average was 3.4. The latter probably would have been greater had all the grades for his premedical courses as well as those studied in graduate school been included. Through an administrative error, the transcript from his graduate school was not received or, by mistake, not put in the applicant's folder. His percentile scores in the MCAT were 99 in the verbal, general information, and science and 85 in the quantitative section.

The applicant is serious about his interest in medicine, pointing out that a physician with a background in sociology can help with the planning and organization of health care. He does not want to be a full-time practitioner of clinical medicine. Although he is attracted to the medical school at which he is being interviewed, in part because of its proximity to a school of public health, he does not want an academic affiliation in the future. In his words, "I find that a scholarly career of teaching and research and pursuit of knowledge for its own sake lacks what is to me a very important component. I feel very strongly a need to be involved in the application of knowledge to human ends."

The temptation to provoke the applicant, but gently, is irresistible. Here is a man with an eleven-year stint as a student-scholar—not a practitioner, doer, or earner of bread. How does he correlate his statement about helping people with his long-term pursuit of learning? How did he finance this leisurely learning? He had received a fellowship for part of the time but also had been supported by his father, a physician associated with a health insurance plan. His mother is also a physician but did not practice medicine since coming to this country because of insufficient training.

Mr. Ross is good natured, intelligent, and seriously interested in medicine in the context of sociological applications. He has the ability and personality to pursue such a course. He probably will not be involved with caring for patients on a one-to-one basis because his interest in tasks completed at a desk seems stronger. This is not the first time that he applied to medical school and it will not be the last time if he fails to get accepted this year because he wants to, and must, achieve his goal. Mr. Ross attended another school.

38.

In this day of keen competition among applicants to medical school, one seeks individuals who will not only be safe in the sense of being able to complete the course but also will make a contribution either to medical knowledge or to the practice of medicine. Attention is paid to the applicant's scholastic achievements, legitimate extracurricular activities, test scores, recommendations, and clues to emotional stability. Consideration of physical attributes or their absence should not enter the equation if objectivity is the goal. However, in describing Lisa Mendel, a 21-year-old applicant from a large university, it would be foolish not to say that she is attractive from all standpoints.

Ms. Mendel is one of seven children, all of whom are normal—and, she adds, all of them are smart. Her major is genetics and her grade point average in science was 4.0 with a cumulative average of 3.8. Her percentile scores on the MCAT were verbal 97, quantitative 95, general information 87, and science 99. She makes abundantly clear the fact that she is interested in the clinical care of patients and not in research. Indeed, one of the reasons she had done research during a summer at the National Cancer Institute was to establish that her interest was in medical practice and not laboratory work. During an earlier summer she worked on a project in marine biology.

Ms. Mendel has taught art voluntarily to school children and has been an academic advisor to students applying for admission to college. Serving as a nurse's aid has strengthened her desire to help people. In answer to a question about what interests her most she says that things that are new to her are interesting.

The applicant has enjoyed meeting medical students and also some of the people working in one of the laboratories in the school at which she is being interviewed. She recognizes the advantages of studying at a medical school that encourages independent study rather than competition among students. Ms. Mendel—bright, self-assured but not overbearing—was accepted by every medical school to which she applied. She enrolled in the school that de-emphasized frequent examinations.

39. James Brown, 21-years-old and neatly presentable, will receive the Bachelor of Science degree in biomedical science after three years of study at an eastern university. His cumulative grade point average and that in science were solidly B+, each being 3.5; his percentile scores on the four sections of the MCAT were 95 except for a 92 in the verbal.

Mr. Brown has already been accepted by four medical schools: one in the Midwest and three in a large city in the East. However, he spontaneously declares that his first choice is the school at which he is being interviewed. Why? As a child he visited the university with his father for football games; he knows students in the undergraduate college and in the medical school and is familiar with the program at the medical school; and, of all the schools he has visited, he likes this school the most of all.

Mr. Brown is relaxed and pleasant as he describes his goal of pursuing a combined career in research and clinical work—perhaps doing research that is related to clinical problems—with some teaching responsibilities while being located at a medical school. He is not interested in private practice. Although he wants a PhD as well as a medical degree, his interest in medicine is stronger than his desire to get a nonmedical doctorate. Indeed, at the end of an hour-long interview, he asks what the interviewer thinks about doing research without working toward a graduate degree. Could one do research that would be useful and also satisfy the requirement of a thesis? Yes, one could. The interviewer thought that Mr. Brown might have asked that question because of his knowledge of the requirement of a thesis for graduation from the medical school and also, perhaps, because of curiosity about doing useful research.

Mr. Brown has carried out two projects for honors. One represented collection of data on public health; namely, validation of death certificates. Another consisted of testing the effects of hormones and drugs on formation of glucose in hepatic cells of rats. The applicant's extracurricular activities consist of his being captain of the college's varsity tennis team, a winner of table tennis, and a participant in bridge and chess tournaments. He also serves as a counselor to students. He has had no experience working in a hospital.

Mr. Brown believes that the school he is visiting is the right place at which to combine graduate and medical work. He was accepted by both the graduate school and the medical school and was offered a place in the combined Medical Scientist Training Program. Mr. Brown, however, enrolled at another school where he will be working only for the medical degree.

40. Dale Lilton is a neatly dressed, slender young

woman of 23 who is thoughtful, friendly, and eager—she arrived a half hour earlier than the scheduled time. She obtained a Bachelor of Arts degree in psychology after three years of study at a state university and then enrolled in a graduate program in clinical psychology. Of interest is the fact that her father is a physician; the daughter had, for a time, rejected his calling. After a year of graduate work the daughter, who has had a lifelong familiarity with medicine, realized that she wanted to do what her father was doing. He loved his work in a clinical pediatric group. And she recognized that although she might have once rebelled against him and his professional choice, a career in medicine was her goal.

Ms. Lilton has been interested in natural science since an early age and her father contributed to that interest when he gave her an inexpensive microscope when she was a child. At that time she looked at leaves and other objects, inspired by Leeuwenhoek. She remembers her excitement in reading the book *Microbe Hunters*. Her main interest is in clinical practice, perhaps with children, and perhaps combined with research. She is considering a future in psychiatry or neuroscience.

The applicant, who is married to a man who intends to be a writer, worked for two years as a volunteer, teaching in a school for autistic children. She also worked at a behavioral clinic for children and in a clinic for parents of autistic children. She was a tutor for Head Start and did research at a psychiatric hospital during one summer, testing the response of patients with schizophrenia to rewards for certain behavioral patterns.

One of the provocative events that influenced her decision to get medical training rather than to continue with graduate work in psychology was the refusal of a senior person at the hospital where she was employed to recommend a general medical workup on a six-year-old child who was considered normal except for his emotional difficulties that were attributed to his parents' behavior. Ms. Lilton thought the child needed a medical workup because he might have been suffering from an illness caused by a known metabolic disorder. She considered that experience one of mistreatment by neglect.

Ms. Lilton's early academic experience at college was not auspicious: her grade point average for the first semester was 2.6. After that her averages for each semester soared, reaching and remaining at 4.0. Following her year of graduate study and work, she returned to college as an undergraduate to study science. She took more than the required premedical courses and earned a grade point average, both cumulative and in science, of 3.7. Her percentile scores on the MCAT were verbal 94, quantitative 74, general information 87, and science 98. Her recommendations are superb. In addition to the volunteer work described, she served as an associate editor of a journal in the behavioral sciences and gave art classes at a state home for girls.

Ms. Lilton is a fine candidate. She is bright and completely motivated toward a career in medicine. Because of the great number of highly qualified applicants, she was put on a waiting list. She attended another school.

41. John Sanders is a pleasant man of 21 who is capable, altruistic, and intelligent but not brilliant. He is majoring in environmental biology at an excellent private university and has earned top-notch grades. His cumulative grade point average at the end of his junior year was over 3.9 with his average in science being 4.0. He has taken the required premedical courses in chemistry and physics and has received advanced placement credit for calculus in high school. Other subjects studied, for which he has received grades of A or Pass—and one B—include psychology and single courses in anthropology, urban studies, art history, music, and general and American literature. In progress are a course in economics and one on the social and psychological origins of disease. He is looking forward to taking a course in health care during the next semester. At the time of the interview he has 21 letter grades and four indicated Pass. His program of study has been a general one and not scholarly in any one subject. Mr. Sanders is consistent—his scores on the MCAT were all in the 90th percentile: verbal 95, quantitative 92, general information 95, and science 96.

Mr. Sanders worked on a laboratory project in a clinical department on alterations in respiration at the cellular level after induced nephrogenic shock in rats and cats. He is not interested in doing research because of his strong interest in clinical care. Indeed, he comes through as a thoroughly selfless person. For example, he intended initially to use the results of his research project as the basis for an honors thesis but decided not to because he does not believe that honors such as summa cum laude or magna cum laude are important. What he does believe in is taking care of patients. He has a strong commitment to community health care in the form of practice and not in the guise of administrative work. He does not like the idea of going into medicine to make money because he does not want to profit from somebody's ill health. He means that. He would not use the term *socialized medicine* because that expression might be anathema to some, but he does want equality of care and an increased distribution to people who do not have medical care. He can see himself practicing medicine in a group but, again, not for profit. He has had some experience helping people by taking part in a program headed by a social worker who makes weekly visits to a boarding home for individuals who previously had been isolated in hospitals or other institutions for the mentally ill. Other activities include working each summer as a truck driver, maintenance man, or agricultural inspector. He keeps up with current events by reading the Sunday newspaper and listening to the radio. And he likes to visit art museums and play the piano. His recommendations are enthusiastic.

The applicant does not have a specific choice of specialization in the broad field of medicine nor is he expected to have one. But he has a particular interest in urban problems and hence in some form of community medical work. He is a very good candidate and was put on a waiting list. He enrolled in the medical school of the university at which he did his undergraduate work.

42.

Susan Leeds is an unusual candidate: intelligent and pleasant, as are most applicants; easy to talk with, as are many applicants; and a holder of an impeccable and interesting academic record. At age 20, as a scholarship student, she is completing four years of schooling at a state university with a major in biochemistry, far more than the required premedical courses in biology and physics and intensive study of several languages: Spanish, Portuguese, French, and German. She also has studied mathematics and has taken single courses in history, anthropology, and music. Her grade point average, both cumulative and in science, was over 3.7; her percentile scores on the MCAT were verbal 88, quantitative 92, general information 83, and science 91. Her university sponsored an educational program abroad and Ms. Leeds was able to study at a European university where her concentration was in biochemistry and genetics. Previously, at her home school, she had worked as a laboratory technician. Upon return she was able to carry out an independent project in immunology. Her stated goal is to enter an MD-PhD program that includes molecular biology because of her interest in the relationship between viruses and cancer.

Another interest is conservation and for a period she worked ten to fifteen hours a week as president of a conservation club. She took part in a tutorial program for three hours a week during one quarter of her first year in college and served as a volunteer at a child care center during part of one summer. The exact input of these activities is not known, although the applicant says that she cut down on them while concentrating on science courses.

Ms. Leeds seems to have a serious interest in basic research and in acquiring a medical background in order to gain a broader point of view. She does not want to get a PhD degree without the medical degree and says that she wants to attend the medical school at which she is being interviewed even if not accepted into the PhD program. Her recommendations are excellent with such words as *intelligence, initiative, spirit,* and *maturity* standing out.

The applicant was not accepted into the graduate school as readily as she was to the medical school because the committee for the former thought she was not as outstanding as their other candidates. Before long, however, she had been accepted by both. What did she do? Ms. Leeds opted for a school without the combined MD-PhD program.

43. Since childhood Brian Patterson, age 21, has thought about human biology. As a result of long discussions with his teacher of physics in high school he became interested in biological applications of physics and is majoring in biophysics at a southern university. As an undergraduate he is doing research in crystallography on projects involving sickle cells and hemoglobin. He feels that the experience in the laboratory has been valuable not just because of the opportunity to study and use several biophysical techniques—such as electron microscopy, X-ray diffraction, column chromatography, and various types of electrophoresis—but more significantly, because he is learning the importance of open mindedness, objectivity, perseverance, ingenuity, and organization in whatever field one enters.

Mr. Patterson is fascinated by neuropathways and functions of the brain and thinks he might want to do clinical work in neurology. He also is interested in research but not in getting a PhD degree. He says, ''I am interested in human beings.'' His familiarity with medicine is based on extended relations with musicians who are physicians. He himself plays first violin in his college's symphony orchestra, serves as concert master, and plays solo clarinet in a two-college band; he is a member of a semiprofessional chamber orchestra. One summer when he thought he might do volunteer work in a hospital he got a job cleaning carpets because he needed the money. For recreation he plays squash racquets and softball and also wrestles.

Mr. Patterson is a serious, quiet young man who does not initiate conversation. Nor is he visibly tense. Being a doctor is important to him. He was recommended highly by the premedical committee at his university; one professor went so far as to say that of the fifty graduate, undergraduate, and postgraduate students he had known in the laboratory during twenty years, the applicant ranked among the top five.

The applicant is bright and capable with a clear talent in music and a strong motivation for medicine. His grade point average, both cumulative and in science, was 3.3. His percentile scores on the MCAT were verbal 47, quantitative 78, general information 38, and science 89. The committee at the school at which he was being interviewed considered him a good candidate but not outstanding in comparison with many other applicants. Mr. Patterson attended a medical school in his home state.

44. Betty Mason, age 20, a pleasant, direct-speaking woman has done exceedingly well in college but not well on the MCAT. Her percentile scores on the latter were verbal 58, quantitative 61, general information 33, and science 84. She is majoring in biology at a state university from which she will receive her Bachelor of Arts degree summa cum laude. Her cumulative grade point average was 3.9 and that in science was 3.89. Her initial desire was to become a veterinarian and during high school she had enrolled in an agricultural course that enabled her to work on a farm and observe the duties of a rural veterinarian. That experience also introduced her to the inadequate health care available to people in the rural community and influenced her decision to become a physician.

During college she has worked as a volunteer in a hospital seeing patients with cardiac and psychiatric problems and also has helped in an emergency room. As a laboratory technician, she has worked in several clinics administered by the department of health in a large city. During the summers she has earned money as a switchboard operator and a receptionist in private companies.

The interviewer asked Ms. Mason what she would like to do more than anything else, exclusive of going to medical school. Ms. Mason answered, "Finish my projects." She has been involved with laboratory research on the effects of temperature and transplantation of organs in insects. She plans to begin a project evaluating the effectiveness of delivery of health care and the satisfaction of the patients, attending a city clinic for venereal disease in comparison with health care and satisfaction of patients being treated in private practice.

Other activities include voluntarily teaching disadvantaged students two or three times a week, horseback riding, ballet dancing, playing the guitar, and reading *Scientific American* and fiction. Her recommendations are enthusiastic throughout with emphasis on her intelligence, motivation, and personality.

Ms. Mason's goal is to practice medicine, possibly cardiology. She wants to take care of patients in an academic environment in which teaching is possible. She was interviewed by two people: one strongly supported her application, the other insisted that under no circumstances should she be admitted because she was naive in thinking that she could go to offices of physicians in private practice and interview their patients being treated for venereal disease. It is only fair to say that the candidate had made it clear that the way would be opened for her by an advisor in the city health department. The insistence on her rejection could not be overcome. Ms. Mason enrolled in another school.

45. Giles Redmon, age 21, is a bright, agreeable, straightforward young man whose predominant interest is in the clinical practice of internal medicine. He expresses admiration for his father, a chemist who enabled his son to acquire a scientific outlook. And the son intends to emulate his father's teaching him to question things as they are but will follow the path of the family's physician who practices internal medicine and is affiliated with a hospital.

Mr. Redmon is mature as well as pleasant and has strong feelings of responsibility. He recently married a girl whom he has been friends with since the first year of high school. She is training to become a teacher. He has been working during the school year grading about 250 papers in chemistry every week, and, during the summers, working as a house painter and as a director of a day camp for children, in order to finance their marriage.

He is attending a fine private university and will receive a Bachelor of Arts degree in biochemistry after four years of study. He will be graduated with honors because his grade point averages, both cumulative and in science, were 3.5, equivalent to B+. His achievement on the MCAT was very good with the following percentile scores: verbal 83, quantitative 95, general information 93, and science 93.

The applicant has been carrying out a research project involving the immunization of rabbits with bacteria, measuring the animal's immunologic response and endeavoring to produce antibodies. He is interested in the project, but his future goal is medical practice and not research. He indicates that his academic program of four courses each semester, many of which were in the hard sciences, was heavy enough to prohibit extracurricular activities except those that he could do at a personal level such as playing tennis, volleyball, football, and skiing.

There is no question about Mr. Redmon's intelligence, ability, and motivation for a career in medicine. It is clear that he will be a good doctor and a good family man. Because of the crush of applicants, he was put on a waiting list. He enrolled in another excellent medical school.

46. Sally Mesmer, a 20-year-old student at a private university noted for expertise in science and technology, expects to get her Bachelor of Science degree with a major in biology after three years of study. Her cumulative grade point average was 3.5 and her average in science was 3.2. Those scholastic averages were based on letter grades in eleven courses. Fourteen courses were marked "Pass" — it is the policy of her school not to grade subjects studied during the first year — or were ungraded because they were in progress.

She has not taken the MCAT but plans to take it in the spring just before graduation from college. Hence, the results of that examination will not be available when the admissions committee evaluates her application. She has applied to only one medical school, that at which she is being interviewed. She says that she did not believe the MCAT was necessary for admission to medical school because she thought the school could take other parts of her application into greater consideration.

Ms. Mesmer has been interested in medicine since second grade — first wanting to be a nurse and then a doctor. She did volunteer work in a psychiatric outpatient clinic during one school year, helped work on a patient advocate plan for a large city hospital, was a member of the student-faculty committee to develop the curriculum of the biology department at her school, and served on the college's committee on discipline. In addition, she helped a faculty member advising freshmen about academic and personal problems. She also plays four musical instruments. Other interests include clinical research on ways to provide oxygen to patients suffering from respiratory diseases and a laboratory project in which she studied the cell cycle of an organism useful in research in genetics.

The applicant is an only child. Her mother died of a cardio-respiratory ailment after Ms. Mesmer entered college and her father does not want her to go to medical school but urges her to return to their home in another city. She is strongly motivated to go to medical school and if she were not accepted the first time she would try again the following year. She seems to have had her fill of science and is eager to get on with clinical medicine.

An intelligent, active young woman, the applicant has applied only to one medical school. Why? Because that school is her first choice. She misjudged the requirements for admission to that school. Perhaps she thought that a medical school that provided a flexible program, one without traditional regimentation, would be more likely than other schools to overlook the absence of the Medical College Aptitude Test.

Or perhaps she thought that her enthusiasm and the breadth of her extracurricular activities would compensate for the scholastic shortfall. She was not accepted.

47. Gary Proctor, a not very big young man of 21 years who is easy to talk with and pleasant, is majoring in biology at a private university. His work in college, as reflected by his grades, was ordinary. The cumulative average and that in science were 3.0. Closer inspection of his record, however, showed a C in every course during his freshman year except for one B. In his second and third years there was increasing improvement as indicated by the accumulation of B's and A's. His strength is in biology and not in the physical sciences, mathematics, or the humanities.

It is clear that Mr. Proctor, who earned a high rank in his class at high school, got off to a shaky start in college, but as time went on he adjusted and steadily raised his academic record. Studying independently, he worked on two projects that required library research and received course credit for them. His performance on the MCAT was good with percentile scores of 94, 78, 97, and 89 in the verbal, quantitative, general information, and science sections. He believes that the MCAT measures quick recall of information, requires ability in abstract reasoning, and is a measure of intelligence.

Mr. Proctor is a plugger who works systematically and hopes that his improvement will land him a place in medical school. He has gone about his work in a businesslike way and engaged in extracurricular activities that would demonstrate his high interest in a medical career. He had been told by the premedical committee at his college that working in a hospital — for example, in an emergency room — indicated motivation. In order to gain direct familiarity with medicine he worked as a volunteer transporting patients in a hospital. He also had been a counselor at a summer camp for underprivileged children, worked as a teaching assistant in a biology course, and served as a technician in a research laboratory. Other activities included the chairmanship of an undergraduate curriculum committee, singing with a group, being a member of a ski team, and attending sherry hours during which a foreign language was spoken.

The applicant says that he wants to go to the school that he is visiting because he knows that he would be "reaching." His goal is to practice clinical medicine, possibly one of the surgical specialties. His recommendations are laudatory. He is intelligent and hard working and there is no doubt that he would perform well as a physician. He was not accepted at this school and he enrolled elsewhere.

48. Alan Paré is 21 and an only child of parents who stressed the importance of education. He did well in high school and majored in biology at college, earning a grade point average in science of 4.0 and a cumulative average of 3.8. In addition to the premedical requirements, he studied biochemistry, anthropology, and several courses in the humanities, including English, two semesters of mathematics, and one semester each of art, music appreciation, and a foreign language. The number of courses taken during the four years of college was average. His percentile scores on the MCAT were verbal 24, quantitative 82, general information 48, and science 86. His impression of the MCAT is that it measures how quickly one can work and how much one has memorized.

Mr. Paré has been on the honors list of an eastern university and is a member of four clubs and one musical society. He spent one semester studying the effects of a chemotherapeutic agent on a malignant tumor and is developing an interest in immunology. He plays a musical instrument and during the summer vacations has worked three to four hours a night, six times a week, as a professional musician. During the days he helps around the house, is active in sports, and reads.

The applicant's interest in becoming a physician arose while studying biology in high school. His actual familiarity with medicine is limited, but his motivation for following a medical career is great. His goal is to be a surgeon practicing near home or in a large city hospital. Mr. Paré is friendly and straightforward although perhaps worried. His academic performance in college has been excellent and recommendations from his professors are strong. His scores on the quantitative and science sections of the MCAT, as well as his performance in his college courses, indicate that he will have no trouble in medical school. He comes across as being more hard working than brilliant but he will be a capable physician. At the time of the interview he had been accepted by two medical schools and he eventually enrolled at one of them.

49. Stephen Lister is a 21-year-old eager, well-spoken, highly presentable young man who is majoring in biology at a private university. He has considerable drive and is determined to pursue a career in medicine. If he were not accepted into medical school in the current year, he would continue to take courses and would reapply the next year. He believes in the power of positive thinking: "When I want something, I work for it. And the goal becomes a reality."

Mr. Lister's academic preparation includes, in addition to several courses in biology, the required ones in physics and chemistry plus biochemistry, mathematics, psychology, philosophy, literature, art, and music. His program is similar to that of most premedical students who do not have a strong interest in the hard sciences but fulfill the requirements and round out their undergraduate education with morsels from the humanities. And, like most premedical students, he is bright, capable of hard work, and interested in clinical medicine. His grade point averages, both cumulative and in science, were 3.7; his percentile scores on the MCAT were verbal 88, quantitative 82, general information 94, and science 96.

For three summers the applicant has worked voluntarily and steadfastly on a project in physiology in a hospital laboratory. He expects the work to result in a paper by two physicians and himself. There is no doubt that he found the clinical research interesting. His aim, however, is to be a completely knowledgeable physician based in a hospital where he can care for interesting patients in an environment in which other well-trained physicians will contribute to intellectual stimulation. He seems to have a genuine understanding of what is involved in research and is not sure that he has the creative ability to identify and work on the solution of problems in a laboratory. His forte will be the practice of medicine.

Mr. Lister's enthusiasm is boundless but well controlled and not obnoxious. He answers immediately, and with a glow, when asked to describe a project that he initiated on his own and goes on to discuss an object he built in a woodworking shop. At college he worked with two other students writing a script for a film. Because of lack of money they did not shoot the film but they learned something en route. He was captain of the debate team at college and won an award in debating. He plays chess but not on a competitive team. His recommendations are very good and he himself is an excellent candidate.

Mr. Lister was accepted for admission to the school at which he was being interviewed, but he became a WBA — withdrawal before acceptance — when he withdrew his application before receiving notification of the acceptance.

50. Ms. Evangeline had been described to the interviewer as an older woman with a lifelong desire to become a physician who had been held back because of a deprived background that included poverty, a disinterested family, and a poor education in the public school system. Living as a welfare mother and supporting a seven-year-old child, she worked voluntarily in community projects to help people needier than herself. Always caring, always helping others, and driven by fierce determination, she went through fire (arson perpetrated by a neighbor), water (environmental pollution), and rape at knife point while living in a slum, struggling to obtain the credentials that would make her acceptable to the best of all possible medical schools.

Who is Ms. Evangeline? The interviewer used the title *Ms.*, initiated with the women's movement, inadvisedly because the candidate's devotion to the poor does not permit sympathy for a movement that is not noted for its support among the underprivileged. Ms. Evangeline is a yellow-haired, delicately petite lady of 31 years whose polished speech is smoother than that of an everyday middle-class female.

Her father has been a carpenter and a railroad clerk but is unemployed. Her mother holds a Bachelor of Arts degree and is a school teacher. In high school the applicant did well in languages, music, and biology but "I was not allowed to take chemistry and trigonometry as these were described by the counselors as 'boys' subjects. That was in the fifties when it was still okay for counselors to say things like that."

After completing high school in 1960, she enrolled at the state university not far from her home in the West. She earned A's in first-year German and French and in voice instruction, a B in composition, and C's in piano and dance. "It seemed expected of me that I would continue at the university in music and languages. I talked to my advisors about the premedical course. They laughed right out loud. I thought there must have been something wrong with my thinking, so I took their advice and registered for music and languages. . .I was hounded by three departments (French, German, and voice) to declare majors in their fields. . .I was actively discouraged from trying premed courses, so I left school at 19. I simply didn't have the grit and courage then to follow my own instincts."

While visiting an art museum she saw a one-man show and was so impressed by the work that she fell in love with the unknown artist. Friends introduced her to the artist and romance conquered. They were married and a child was born; man and wife had different interests, so they were divorced but parted as good friends. The child was born in the year preceding the divorce. The father contributes $100 a month to the child's support for nine months of each year.

During the six years of marriage the applicant registered for classes at the state university every other year, "under pressure from family and friends," taking courses similar to those already described as well as more esoteric ones such as Islamic civilization and culture. And every other year she dropped out. She did not study any subjects that might be interpreted as premedical. Her grade point average was 2.3. Several times she enrolled and withdrew for "lack of interest." Her real interests were in direct community work.

During those years of marriage to the painter-sculptor, before there were free medical and mental health clinics, drug dependency units, neighborhood offices for legal assistance, crisis centers, and other agencies to handle day-to-day problems in the community, she served as a self-appointed social worker. She kept lists of physicians, psychologists, "clean" abortionists, lawyers, and landlords who would reduce their customary fees in order to help street people and blacks. She co-sponsored an auction at an art museum; was involved in preservation of a city square and the farmer's market; and raised money for Planned Parenthood, the restoration of paintings damaged in the floods in Florence, the rebuilding of a bombed Sunday school in the South, and for burying the children who had been killed. Other times she raised bail for people who had gone south for Freedom Rights and for drives to register voters. She also served as an assistant to a costumer in a summer theatre.

After her divorce, for three years she worked 24 hours a day as a personal secretary, editorial assistant, and nurse for a writer. The last year of work was in South America where she learned Portuguese and managed her employer's holdings; that is, she oversaw repairs on the employer's house that required attention to electrical circuitry, storm drainage, and installation of the town's first septic tank. By the end of that year she knew without a doubt that she wanted to go home to prepare for the study of medicine and that she "had the grit and confidence necessary to do it."

She applied to, was accepted by, and enrolled in the department of continuing education at a fine college for women in the Northeast in order to study mathematics, physics, and biology. She had no funds of her own and her former employer paid half of her tuition. She secured a bank loan for the balance and applied to welfare in order to survive because she could not be a full-time student and mother and maintain a job as well. She and her child took a room in a private house but had to move after the landlady's child set fire to the living room.

She felt miserable at school. Never before had she seen true-false and multiple-choice examinations — and she "hadn't a clue as to how to prepare for them." She had expected to find an atmosphere of solidarity and trust and had not been prepared for the cutthroat world of premedical education: "I couldn't bear the isolation from the grit and grime of the real world, the sterility of the institution, the endless and meaningless politeness, the uninventive approach to life." She withdrew from the college in the third month only because it was clear that she had made a bad choice of school. She was determined to continue to prepare for medicine. No statement from that college was included in her application to medical school.

During the next two years she was enrolled in an adult education program at a graduate school in which she could be a candidate for a Master of Arts degree in community health planning. The faculty of that school granted her a baccalaureate equivalence to allow her to enter the graduate school. The program included field work in community service and independent reading in the subjects she wanted to study: infant mortality, nutrition, parasitology, and water quality. She earned honors in courses in the biology of women, health planning, medical sociology, nutrition, and introduction to radiation physics—44 credit hours of A.

Some gnawing questions remained with the interviewer: why the circuitous route into graduate school through the back door of the baccalaureate equivalence, jumping into soft courses and easy reading, instead of biology, chemistry, and mathematics at a high school level to prepare for premedical subjects that would provide a genuine learning experience and a base upon which to build after admission to medical school?

One summer during the two years that she attended the graduate school, she studied inorganic chemistry at another university and earned a C-. She challenged the teacher and the grade: the teacher told her that she would never get a grade higher than that from him. In the fall and winter of one of those years and in the spring of the new year, she studied at a different school and received a B in animal biology, C's in physics, and two grades of incomplete in organic chemistry with a grade point average of 2.3. At the same time she was a member of the health advisory corporation for a neighborhood health center in a housing project. She spoke to her organic chemistry teacher about the scheduling of the course. He remarked that she had come on strong, being disturbed because his lectures were at the same time as her meetings at the health clinic. As a result of the conflict, she had lost her seat on the board. The teacher explained that the time of the lectures was the time assigned for that chemistry course.

During the period in which she was trying to study premedical courses at different schools she struggled along on student loans, welfare, and pluck. She and her son lived in a substandard housing project exposed to danger. There she was beaten and raped and the apartment was broken into.

The summer after she had studied inorganic chemistry, and at the same university, she was admitted into a health career program for disadvantaged students. She was given financial aid that enabled her to resign from welfare. Her grades were A- in a tutorial in natural science and B+ in selected topics in cell biology. In the fall she continued as a special student and submitted her applications to medical school.

At the time of her interview she said that she was getting A's in math —a course that included algebra, logarithms, and trigonometry—and that she was also taking a tutorial in organic chemistry in which she would get an A. Her tutor praised the student's extraordinary memory, how she transcribed every single reaction in the first nine chapters of the text onto note cards and committed the whole lot to memory. Her grade was B.

The application showed a grade point average in science of 3.1 for work done at five universities and a cumulative average of 3.5. The MCAT had been taken twice and the higher percentile scores were verbal 94, quantitative 09, general information 73, and science 22.

Recommendations included two letters from the applicant's chief advisor — one letter was of four pages and the other of six, each typed single spaced. Courses were described, in some instances with comments by instructors. The applicant's personal qualities such as understanding the health problems of the poor, dedication to a career, extraordinary ability to communicate, and capacity for hard work were extolled. Although some of the courses had been set up by her advisor, the applicant had not been a student in courses taught by the advisor. In addition there were nine individual recommendations from people who did not know the applicant as a student in class but who knew her because of her work in community health or as an advisee. A letter from a psychologist at the applicant's high school noted that she had a high IQ, was the student who cared for the epileptic students who had seizures in class, and that her teachers encouraged her to study nursing. And then: "We were backward. We should have known that she was meant to be a physician."

The applicant's greatest strength was in supporting the underprivileged. During the time she was at the neighborhood health center she initiated a move to get a microscope for the gynecology clinic and served as a representative on the laboratory committee to discuss improvement in communication of laboratory reports from lab to nurse to doctor to patient. During the year in which she was applying to medical school she worked at a children's hospital on weekends, met informally with community groups to discuss health needs of various sections of the community, and became a laboratory trainee at a free health center to gain skills needed for working in a women's clinic.

The applicant desires to be an evangelist against waste of all forms

— time, space, material, and human resources. How would she go about achieving that well-stated desire? Her primary concern is in the delivery of health care. She would like to direct a community health clinic. Wouldn't that require a lot of administrative work and put distance between herself and the patients? That did not matter because other people would help with the medical care and administrative work while she planned the overall needs of the people. She also is interested in what makes people ill — not in emotional illness or finding the cause of cancer or of heart disease but in diagnosing and treating diseases. She wants to work in a neighborhood that serves the poor. She would not want to treat people of the middle class. Why not? "I do not understand middle-class people or their problems."

Her immediate goal is to get the best possible education at the best possible medical school to become the best possible physician. Her long term goal is to design on a national scale health services for poor urban communities. She would include training programs for residents in the community and house-to-house visits by health workers. She would introduce clinics for screening, computerized information on the immune status of each child with automatic printouts of the names of children due for boosters in the next period, prenatal classes and exercises, discussion groups for diabetics, separate services for adolescents, community vans for transportation of patients to clinics, and voluntary rotation of nurses to care for people who were sick in bed at home. She would design services for prevention and early diagnosis of chronic diseases and for control of infectious diseases. She would include in her national design guidelines for community participation so that people in the neighborhood would not be left out of the decision-making process. People who are left out of decision making feel like victims instead of beneficiaries of health care, especially when members of the professions tell them what to do. But, as pointed out to her by another interviewer, a psychiatrist, she would be a professional herself after completing medical training. And how would the community feel when she told them what to do? She said that she is one of the community, not of the establishment. She knows poverty and she and her ideas would be accepted by the poor. Her goal of aiding the poor is laudable. How would she implement it? She answered that her past experience would help her, that she knew how to deliver health care.

The applicant's worthy aims are not new ones and many have already been put into practice. What new proposals does she have? She says that she is the one who will present new ideas. But she does not have any — none that have not been proposed already.

Her interest in helping is not limited to small problems. In the 1960s she initiated a project that involved petitioning the governor of one state to refuse a request from the governor of another state to extradite a black man accused of a crime. The applicant had heard about the man who was working in a fruit-growing area. The request for extradition had been made because the man, in the course of robbing an attendant in a gasoline station, had murdered him. Since that event the laborer had been doing well, working and so on. The applicant had found out from the American Civil Liberties Union that the governor of the state in which the worker was employed could request reasons for the extradition. Because the governor seeking the extradition did not supply the data, the request for extradition was denied. The applicant had saved the man from extradition. But she did that without knowing him. She had not talked to the man herself. Why not? The applicant answered, ''Why should I?'' The outcome had been excellent. But the savior had not learned anything about the individual for herself. Everything she had done had been a result of hearsay. The psychiatrist felt that she came across in a grandiose manner and that she generated a lot of pressure in a quiet, determined way. That interviewer was similar in age and background to the applicant, had gone to high school at the same time, and was the only one in the high school class to go to college.

The applicant believes that one of the difficulties inherent in the system of medical education is that poor people are hand picked for medical training with encouragement to join the establishment rather than to return to their own communities to practice. The unspoken attitude toward the economically deprived students is "you are special. You can make it. You can have a better life. You can become one of us." Instead, the students could be encouraged to lose their shame of poverty and to work for their own people. If physicians' salaries were limited, a different kind of applicant would receive training, one who would help the poor. Physicians' salaries should be equitable without the patients getting ripped off. She would need only $10,000 per year for herself and her child.

What does she think is the commonest reason for becoming a doctor? "That question cannot be answered." Could she make a guess? "No. Most people have a mixed bag of feelings." About how many people, given a range of zero to one hundred, or a few or a lot, like their jobs? "That question cannot be answered because a lot of people don't know that they don't like their jobs."

The questions were not prompted by the interviewer's trying to discover if the applicant were up to date on social surveys. The interviewer was not familiar with actual studies about motives for becoming a physician or about the extent of job satisfaction in the United States but was seeking direct answers to what seemed like simple, commonsense questions. Could the applicant suggest why the scores on the MCAT went down the second time around except in science? "Did they? I didn't know that." The interviewer responded optimistically, "You probably didn't get to see the results." There was silence, and then the answer, "Yes, I did see them."

There was some follow-up regarding the applicant's early schooling. The transcript from high school showed credit for algebra and plain geometry, courses required for admission to the state university, as well as English, United States history, civics, French, Spanish, biology, but not solid geometry, trigonometry, chemistry, or physics. The interviewer, having lived in the same part of the country that had been home for the applicant, had friends and colleagues in the cities in which the applicant attended high school and the state university. One of them, a member of the clinical faculty of the medical school at the university at which the applicant had first enrolled, was asked for information about the university and the high school that discouraged women from studying mathematics and science in the late 1950s. The friend was surprised, almost to the point of disbelief. He could imagine peer pressure in the high school keeping a girl from taking science courses but not pressure from teachers and counselors.

The interviewer had some direct familiarity with the state university as a result of spending a summer there as a visitor to the medical school at one of the same times that the applicant had been enrolled as an undergraduate. The university is a big one and, as would be expected of a good school, offered an almost limitless range of courses. The professional colleague, who had been a premedical student there almost twenty years before the applicant, and who had gone to a different school for medical training, was asked about the attitudes toward women interested in taking premedical courses. He insisted that the university, in its bigness, was so impersonal that it was impossible for him to believe that anyone would take enough interest in a student, female or male, to encourage or discourage the taking of individual courses. All a student had to do was to go through the school's catalog, pick out courses, and register for them.

It seemed likely that the applicant's talents in voice and languages were significant and that members of the faculty might have encouraged her to select courses in their fields. But it seemed less likely that anyone would have prevented her, or actively discouraged her, from studying premedical subjects in the 1960s. The application was florid, a tour de force. The applicant has had some successes, but the way she rationalizes her failures is enormous. So many excuses were given that the application was beginning to shape up as a put-on, the greatest hoax since the discovery of the skull of Piltdown man.

In summary, the applicant is a physically attractive woman who is relaxed, smooth spoken, altruistic and a little evasive. In the interview she comes across as a one-person crusade. Her goals are laudable. Her ideas for achieving them are nonexistent. It seems unlikely that she will contribute innovations to social change. That is not meant to deny her admission to medical school. In one recommendation from the applicant's chief advisor, she is described as one of the most impressive people the advisor has ever met, one that has a contribution to make to American medicine that can be matched by precious few people. None of the premedical students at the school of the letter-writer could approach the applicant in vision and understanding of poor communities nor in the human qualities that would translate that vision into reality. The advisor wrote, ''She has got real guts.''

The interviewer agrees that the applicant has guts and that she should be permitted to become a physician. The interviewer also hopes that the applicant will matriculate at another school. She did.

Too often in the search for the well-rounded person with wide interests that might indicate that one is not a grind, the individual with unique talent is passed over. Diffusion should not be mistaken for diversity. Nor should community or hospital service be substituted for ability and academic excellence. Admissions committees at medical schools try hard to avoid missing an outstanding candidate. They also don't want to be caught with someone who can't make the grade.

4
Summings Up And The Future Of Medical School Admissions

Factors that Work in Your Favor at the Interview

The interview for admission to medical school is one of the most important events in your planning for the future. In a sense, its significance ranks with writing a will. The interview must be taken seriously but seriousness of purpose does not require elimination of evidence of a sense of humor. Demonstration of wit is welcome as long as the student does not seem superficial or lacking in dedication to a career in medicine.

Arrive for the interview on time or even five minutes early because it might take awhile to find the location of the interview site. If the interviewer is late, try not to let the interviewer know that you have been kept waiting or that you might have had other important things to do. The interviewer may have been late because of seeing patients, giving a lecture, or carrying out a surgical procedure. The chances are that he or she did not forget about you.

It is important to be wide awake and honest and not to exaggerate your extracurricular activities or scholastic achievements. If a worthwhile project has been done in college, be prepared to explain it accurately.

You should have some ideas about what your goals are in medicine. Let the interviewer know that you are interested in practicing medicine.

Do not be afraid to ask the interviewer questions. Some people like to have the applicant show an interest in their academic work.

Do not make disparaging remarks about your college, your instructors, or other students.

Be acquainted with the goals of the medical school at which you are being interviewed and also with the kinds of students who attend that school. No harm is done by acting as if the school at which you are being interviewed is the school that you would like most to attend.

In general, it is better to be interviewed by a member of the admissions committee at the medical school to which you are applying or by a member of that committee who is conducting regional interviews at your school. It is less preferable to be interviewed by an individual who happens to live near your home or college and who is an alumnus or alumna of the medical school to which you are applying, but who is not a member of the admissions committee.

The Applicants

Most of the applicants to medical school are capable and, indeed, well qualified. Some are outstanding. A lesser number could not handle the work load because of emotional problems or poor ability.

No one has done the experiment of selecting a first-year class, or a part of one, from the large group of applicants who were eliminated on the basis of initial screening of their applications. There are undoubtedly many good people who would make very good doctors who did not reach the stage of the interview. What happens to them? Many, but not all, apply the next year to medical schools within or outside of the United States. Some get jobs in hospitals or at medical schools. Others work voluntarily or for stipends in a service-related organization to help bolster their next round of applications. There are those who enroll for training in allied health professions. Graduate work attracts some former premedical students.

The number of applicants expected to apply to medical school for the entering class of 1977 will probably exceed that of 1976. Why are there so may applicants? The stated reasons are many and they are not necessarily put in the order of truth:

1. Other options are closed.
2. The practice of medicine is a good way to earn a living.
3. The practice of medicine is a *very* good way to earn a living.
4. Medicine is one profession that an individual can pursue in an independent fashion. The work load is limited or extended depending on the physician's eagerness and capacity for work. Doctors earn a lot of money if they work hard and satisfy their patients.
5. Prestige. The profession of medicine is a respected one, encompassing as it does the requirements of intelligence, knowledge, understanding, and the chance for nobility.
6. The desire to help people. The opportunity to make a sick person well is great and, in many situations, satisfying.
7. Intellectual fulfillment. Entering the field of medicine simply for the learning experience or as a solution to one's personal problems is not a valid aim although some applicants have indicated that as their goal.
8. Interest in the subject matter. The subject of medicine is the human being. And the field of medicine is a fascinating one in which there is continually new knowledge that the good physician strives to absorb. The challenges of making an innovation in a procedure or a treatment or, most exciting of all, in furthering the understanding of a disease are unlimited.

There are many roles to play in medicine and many places to perform them. Most of the roles and places do not require scientific stars. Ten to twenty years ago premedical students said they wanted to be doctors because of their interest in science. In the 1970s the commonest reason given for wanting to become a doctor is to serve people.

For tomorrow? One expects that there will be a surplus of physicians in the next decade as a result of the expanded training of primary care physicians, nurse practitioners, and physicians' assistants. There should be a better distribution of medical care because of the continuing increase in well-trained medical helpers but we do not know if that will happen. One also expects that the numbers of applicants to medical school will continue to soar.

At the new medical school of Ben Gurion University, situated in a part of the world in which there is a crying need for physicians to provide primary care in a desert, students are selected not on the basis of scores in a medical college admission test nor on a cumulative grade point average but on the basis of proved excellence in any two academic subjects out of five or six national matriculation examinations. That kind of performance indicates that the student is capable of adequate achievement when interested and motivated. If the student were intelligent enough and hard-working enough to do well in two scholastic endeavors, the student would be capable of becoming a physician. In addition the personal characteristics of the applicant — his or her attitudes and values — are determined during an hour-long interview with a two-person team of interviewers. Psychometric tests are also given. The qualities sought in the prospective physician, in addition to intelligence, are integrity, humility, empathy, stability, enthusiasm, intellectual flexibility, capacity for cooperation, ability to admit when wrong, desire to assume responsibility, capacity for self-learning, and interest in service to the community.

Because of the great number of men and women applying to medical schools in the United States, what might be a fairer method of accepting a first-year class than the procedures followed today? One possibility that would give every applicant an equal chance would be a lottery. That procedure, by eliminating the interview, would certainly cut down the work for members of admissions committees. Another suggestion, made by Dr. Edmund D. Pellegrino, a medical educator and professor of medicine, would be to select the entering class by choosing applicants from three categories.

Group I   Fifteen percent of the prospective class: cumulative grade point average 3.8 to 4.0 with scores in the Medical College Admission Test in the 90th percentile. An interview would be required. The individuals selected would be the academic type with high ability in science as well as in other subjects.

Group II   Seventy percent of the class: cumulative grade point average 3.2 to 3.79 with scores in the MCAT in the 80th percentile. Selection would be based on a lottery without any interview.

Group III   Fifteen percent of the class: cumulative grade point average 2.67 to 3.2 with scores in the MCAT in the 70th percentile. An interview would be required to discover their assets.

The first group might consist of the innovators. The second group would be made up of highly motivated, hard-working people who would enter the clinical specialties or family medicine. The third group would be those whose strengths consisted of high motivation and humane qualities that could not be found in grade point averages and test scores.

For today? The applicant to medical school should get good grades, do well in the MCAT, get to know the teachers of his or her college courses so that letters of recommendation will be forthcoming, and, if lucky enough to get an interview at a medical school, be as forthright, honest, and appealing as possible.

CHAPTER

5

Applicants, Applications, And Enrollments

Trends in Applications and Enrollments

In 1909, when Abraham Flexner began his on-the-spot study of medical schools in the United States and Canada, there were 150 medical schools in the United States. Many of them were of poor quality. Fifteen years later that number had been reduced by one half.

Between 1914 and 1915 there were 96 medical schools in the United States with a total enrollment of 14,891 of whom 4 percent were women. Although the number of schools had decreased, the number of students increased so that between 1929 and 1930 there were 21,597 students in 76 schools with 4.4 percent of them being women. In the years 1939 to 1940 there were 21,271 students in 77 schools with 5.4 percent of them being women. In 1949 to 1950 there were 79 medical schools with a total enrollment of 25,103 students of whom 7.2 percent were women. The number of female students had increased slowly from 4 percent of all medical students in 1914 to 7.2 percent in 1949. In 1950, 10.7 percent of the graduates from medical school were women. In the years 1954 to 1955, 28,583 students were enrolled in 81 medical schools and the percentage of women fell to 5.4. In 1955 the percentage of female graduates was 4.9. The large number of women enrolled in medical school in the 1940s and graduated from medical school in 1950 undoubtedly reflected the admission of more women when men were being called to military service.

In the years 1959 to 1960 there were 85 medical schools with a total enrollment of 30,084 students, 5.7 percent of whom were women; the percentage of female graduates in 1960 also was 5.7. In 1969 to 1970 there were 101 medical schools and 24,465 applicants filing 133,822

Entering Year	1914-15	1929-30	1939-40	1949-50	1954-55
Number of schools	96	76	77	79	81
Number of applicants		13,655	11,800	24,434	14,538
Total acceptances		7,035	6,218	7,150	7,878
% total acceptances		51.5	52.7	29.3	54.2
First-year places		6,457	5,794	7,042	7,576
Number of applications		31,749	34,871	88,244	47,568
Applications per person		2.3	3.0	3.6	3.3
Applications per man			3.0		3.1
Applications per woman			2.4		3.4
% of women of all applicants		3.5	5.4	5.7	6.2
% women accepted of women applicants		65.5	50.8	28.8	52.9
% women accepted of all acceptees		4.5	5.1	5.5	6.0
% women in first-year class		4.5	5.1	5.6	5.9
% men accepted		51.0	52.7	29.3	54.3
Total enrollment	14,891	21,597	21,271	25,103	28,583
% women total enrollment	4.0	4.4	5.4	7.2	5.4
% women graduated	2.6	4.5	5.0	10.7	4.9

* Estimated figures.

†Based on data compiled by W.F. Dubé et al., and published in the *Journal of Medical Education:* Volumes 48 (186-189), 48 (395-420), 49 (1070-1072), 50 (303-306), and 51 (144-146). Data reprinted by permission of W.F. Dubé, Association of American Medical Colleges.

applications, an average of 5.5 each, for the 10,422 places in the first-year class. Women represented 9.4 percent of the applicants and 9.1 percent of the entering class. The total enrollment that year was 37,690 of whom 9 percent were women. Before 1969, with the exception of the years encompassing World War II, the percentage of female medical students remained small. "The percentage of women in first-year classes of all United Stated medical schools has approximated the proportion of women applicants in the period since 1929-30."[1] The number of female applicants increased slowly from 3.5 percent in 1929 to 9.4 percent in 1969.

Table 1
Applicants, Applications, and Enrollments†

1959-60	1969-70	1970-71	1971-72	1972-73	1973-74	1974-75	1975-76
85	101	102	108	114	114	114	114
14,952	24,465	24,987	29,172	36,135	40,506	42,624	43,303
8,512	10,547	11,500	12,335	13,757	14,335	15,066	15,365
56.9	43.1	46.0	42.3	38.1	35.4	35.3	35.5
8,173	10,422	11,348	12,361	13,677	14,159	14,763	15,295
57,888	133,822	148,797	210,943	267,306	328,275	362,376	366,000*
3.9	5.5	6.0	7.2	7.4	8.1	8.5	8.6*
2.6	5.5	6.0	7.3	7.5	8.2	8.5	
2.9	4.8	5.3	6.5	7.1	7.8	8.4	
6.9	9.4	10.9	12.8	15.2	17.8	20.4	22.6*
53.0	44.2	47.4	45.1	43.0	39.5	38.9	38.0*
6.4	9.5	11.2	13.7	17.1	20.0	23.0	23.8*
6.2	9.1	11.1	13.7	166.8	19.7	22.2	23.8
57.2	43.0	45.9	41.9	37.2	34.5	34.4	35.6*
30,084	37,690	40,238	43,650	47,366	50,716	53,554	55,818
5.7	9.0	9.6	10.9	12.8	15.4	18.0	20.5
5.7	8.4	9.2	9.0	8.9	11.1	13.4	

Figure 1
The Number of Applicants,
1969 to 1975

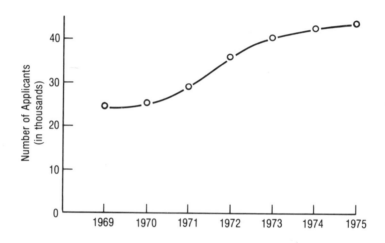

From 1970 to 1971 there were 102 schools to which 24,987 applicants submitted 148,797 applications, an average of 6 each, for 11,348 places in the first-year class. Women represented 10.9 percent of the applicants and 11.1 percent of the first-year class. The total enrollment was 40,238, 9.6 percent being women.

From 1971 to 1972 there were 108 schools and 29,172 applicants filing 210,943 applications, an average of 7.2 each, for 12,361 places in the first-year class. The total enrollment was 43,650 of which 10.9 percent were women. They made up 12.8 percent of the applicants and 13.7 percent of the entering class.[2]

From 1972 to 1973 there were 114 schools and 36,135 applicants submitting 267,306 applications, an average of 7.4 each, for 13,677 places in the first-year class. Women represented 15.2 percent of the

Figure 2
Changes in Percent of Applicants in Successive Years

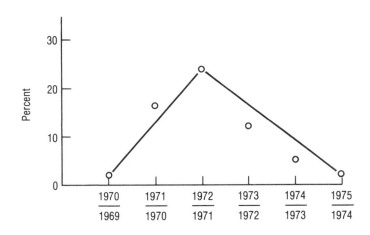

applicants and 16.8 percent of the entering class. The total enrollment was 47,366 of which 12.8 percent were women.

From 1973 to 1974 there were 114 medical schools and 40,506 applicants filing 328,275 applications, an average of 8 each, for 14,159 places in the first-year class. Women represented 17.8 percent of the applicants and 19.7 percent of the entering class. The total enrollment was 50,716, 15.4 percent being women.

Between 1970 and 1973 the applications to medical school doubled. Although the number of applicants for 1973 exceeded the number for 1972 by 4,371 individuals, the annual rate of increase declined. Since 1969, annual percentage increases peaked in 1972 for applicants (24 percent over 1971) and in 1971 for applications (42 percent over 1970). Comparable rates of increases for 1973 amounted

**Figure 3
Number of Applications,
1969 to 1975**

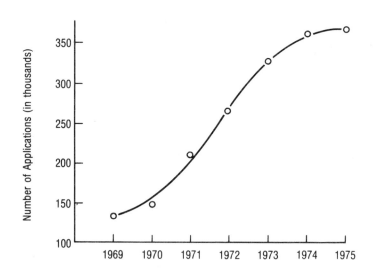

to 12 percent for individuals and 23 percent for applications. The number of applicants and of applications continues to rise yearly, but the rates of increase each year are declining.

Of the 40,506 applicants to the 1973 entering class, 14,335 (35 percent) were accepted (578 or 4 percent more than in 1972) and 13,771 matriculated in United States medical schools for the first time. Repeating, re-entering and advanced standing admission students brought the first year total to 14,124, a gain of 447 (3 percent) over the previous year. The 13,771 new entrants (97 percent of the 1973 first-year total) also increased 3 percent over the previous year (419), but this increase was only one-third of the new entrant gain of 1,264 recorded for 1972.[3]

Figure 4
Changes in Percent of Applications in Successive Years

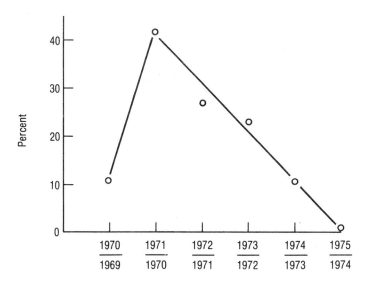

The participation of women in first-year classes was greater in 1974-75 than ever before in the history of U.S. medical education, with 3,275 (22 percent) of all entering class places filled by women . . . and the percentage of matriculants who are women continues to surpass the percentage of applicants who are women. Women accounted for 20 percent of the 1974-75 applicant pool.[4]

Of the total number of women in the first-year class, 17.2 percent are members of a minority group.[5]

In the first-year class of 1974 to 1975, 1,839 students (13 percent) identified themselves as members of a minority group: Black American, Native American, Mexican American, Puerto Rican-Mainland,

and Asian American. In previous years fewer schools were listed for enrolling members of the underrepresented minorities. The number of Black Americans in the entering classes beginning in 1970-71 was 697 (6.1 percent); 1971-72: 882 (7.1 percent); 1972-73: 957 (7.0 percent); 1973-74: 1,027 (7.2 percent); 1974-75: 1,106 (7.5 percent); 1975-76: 1,038 (6.8 percent).

The enrollment of minority students in the first-year class, exclusive of black Americans but including Native Americans, Mexican Americans, Puerto Rican-Mainland, and Asian Americans was as follows: 1970-71: 301 (2.6 percent); 1971-72: 398 (3.3 percent); 1972-73: 480 (3.5 percent); 1973-74: 604 (4.3 percent); 1974-75: 733 (5 percent); 1975-76: 751 (4.9 percent). In the entering class of 1974-75, the largest numerical increase (83) occurred in the black American group and the largest percentage increases (61.4) in the Native American group.

Table 2
First-Year U.S. Minority Student Enrollments†

Groups	1970-71 No.	%	1971-72 No.	%	1972-73 No.	%	1973-74 No.	%	1974-75 No.	%	1975-76 No.	%
Black American	697	6.1	882	7.1	957	7.0	1,027	7.2	1,106	7.5	1,036	6.8
Other Minorities*	301	2.6	398	3.3	480	3.5	604	4.3	733	5.	751	4.9
Total U.S. Minorities	998	8.7	1,280	10.4	1,437	10.5	1,631	11.5	1,839	12.5	1,787	11.7

*Native American, Mexican American, Puerto Rican-Mainland, Asian American.
†Based on date compiled by W.F. Dube and T.L. Gordon and published in the *Journal of Medical Education,* Volume 50 (303-306) and 51 (144-146). Data reprinted by permission of W.F. Dubé, Association of American Medical Colleges.

Table 3
Total U.S. Minority Student Enrollments†

Groups	1970-71 No.	%	1971-72 No.	%	1972-73 No.	%	1973-74 No.	%	1974-75 No.	%	1975-76 No.	%
Black American	1,509	3.8	2,055	4.7	2,582	5.4	3,049	6.0	3,355	6.3	3,456	6.2
Other Minorities*	785	1.9	1,017	2.4	1,336	2.9	1,791	3.5	2,205	4.1	2,472	4.4
Total U.S. Minorities	2,294	5.7	3,072	7.1	3,918	8.3	4,840	9.5	5,560	10.4	5,928	10.6

*Native American, Mexican American, Puerto Rican-Mainland, Asian American.

†Based on data compiled by W.F. Dube and T.L. Gordon and published in the *Journal of Medical Education,* Volume 50 (303-306) and 51 (144-146). Data reprinted by permission of W.F. Dubé, Association of American Medical Colleges.

The total United States minority student enrollment from 1970-1976 was as follows: 1970-71: 2,294 (5.7 percent); 1971-72: 3,072 (7.1 percent); 1972-73: 3,917 (8.3 percent); 1973-74: 4,840 (9.5 percent); 1974-75: 5,560 (10.4 percent); 1975-76: 5,928 (10.6 percent).[6]

6
The Flexner Report

At their meeting in November, 1908, the trustees of the Carnegie Foundation authorized a study and report about the schools of medicine and law in the United States. The study of medical schools was carried out by Abraham Flexner.[1] Before his report "the organization of medical education in this country has hitherto been such as not only to commercialize the process of education itself, but also to obscure in the minds of the public any discrimination between the well trained physician and the physician who has had no adequate training whatsoever."[2] There were no general requirements for admission to medical school; except for a few institutions, students were not selected with much care.

Mr. Flexner began his pilgrimage in 1909 and for some three or four years devoted himself to observation of medical schools in this country and in western Europe. His critical report to the Carnegie Foundation in 1910 was responsible for the transformation of medical schools in the United States from, in many cases, diploma mills to outstanding institutions of learning and research. When he began his odyssey "there were one hundred and fifty-odd schools, so-called, in this country . . . . " Fifteen years later "that number had been practically cut in half."[3]

In order to improve medical education it was necessary to improve both secondary and college education regarding scholarship and to have the universities play a role: "to a considerable, though varying extent, clinical teaching continues to be an incident in the life of a busy practitioner. The good practitioner is, and should be, the busy practitioner; the teacher, however, needs leisure to investigate. The two callings are inherently at war. . . . ''[4]

As a result of the report, low-grade professional schools that universities maintained only for their ''institutional completeness'' were eliminated and university standards of scholarship were extended into the medical school so that the study of medicine could become an intellectual pursuit. The curriculum in which preclinical sciences preceded clinical subjects was inaugurated. ''The teachers of the laboratory branches and . . . [the] clinical teachers . . . interested in the study of disease, want a solid foundation for their instruction.''[5]

In 1924 Mr. Flexner pointed out that the progress in this country was quicker and greater than anywhere else because we had further to go; the differences between good and bad were more marked than in any other country in the western world. He credited the progress to leaders in the profession and the schools and the Council of Medical Education of the American Medical Association.[6]

Medical Schools in the United States and their Dates of Organization

1765   University of Pennsylvania School of Medicine, Philadelphia
1767   Columbia University College of Physicians and Surgeons, New York
1783   Harvard Medical School, Boston
1797   Dartmouth Medical School, Hanover
1807   University of Maryland School of Medicine, Baltimore
1812   Yale University School of Medicine, New Haven
1819   University of Cincinnati College of Medicine, Cincinnati
1822   University of Vermont College of Medicine, Burlington
1823   Medical University of South Carolina College of Medicine, Charleston
1824   Jefferson Medical College of Thomas Jefferson University, Philadelphia

1825 George Washington University School of Medicine, Washington, D.C.

1825 University of Virginia School of Medicine, Charlottesville

1828 Medical College of Georgia, Augusta

1834 Tulane University School of Medicine, New Orleans

1834 State University of New York College of Medicine, Syracuse

1837 University of Louisville School of Medicine, Louisville

1838 Medical College of Virginia, Richmond

1839 Albany Medical College of Union University, Albany

1840 University of Missouri School of Medicine, Columbia

1841 New York University School of Medicine, New York

1843 Case Western Reserve University School of Medicine, Cleveland

1846 State University of New York at Buffalo

1848 Hahneman Medical College and Hospital, Philadelphia

1850 Medical College of Pennsylvania (formerly Woman's), Philadelphia

1850 University of Iowa College of Medicine, Iowa City

1850 University of Michigan Medical School, Ann Arbor

1851 Georgetown University School of Medicine, Washington, D.C.

1851 University of Tennessee College of Medicine, Memphis

1854 Emory University School of Medicine, Atlanta

1859 University of Alabama School of Medicine, Birmingham

1859 Northwestern University School of Medicine, Chicago

1860 New York Medical College, New York

1860 State University of New York College of Medicine, Brooklyn

1864 University of California School of Medicine, San Francisco

1868 Howard University College of Medicine, Washington, D.C.

1873 Boston University School of Medicine, Boston

1873 Vanderbilt University School of Medicine, Nashville

1876 Meharry Medical College School of Medicine, Nashville

1879 University of Arkansas School of Medicine, Little Rock

1879 University of North Carolina School of Medicine, Chapel Hill

1881 University of Illinois College of Medicine, Chicago
1881 University of Nebraska College of Medicine, Omaha
1883 University of Colorado School of Medicine, Denver
1883 University of Minnesota Medical School, Minneapolis
1883 University of Pittsburgh School of Medicine, Pittsburgh
1885 Wayne State University School of Medicine, Detroit
1885 University of Southern California School of Medicine, Los Angeles
1887 University of Oregon Medical School, Portland
1887 University of Texas Medical Branch, Galveston
1892 Creighton University School of Medicine, Omaha
1893 Johns Hopkins University School of Medicine, Baltimore
1893 Tufts University School of Medicine, Boston
1898 Cornell University Medical College, New York
1899 Washington University School of Medicine, St. Louis
1900 Baylor College of Medicine, Houston
1900 University of Oklahoma School of Medicine, Oklahoma City
1901 Temple University School of Medicine, Philadelphia
1902 Bowman Gray School of Medicine, Winston-Salem
1902 West Virginia University School of Medicine, Morgantown
1903 Indiana University School of Medicine, Indianapolis
1903 St. Louis University School of Medicine, St. Louis
1903 University of Mississippi School of Medicine, Jackson
1905 University of Kansas School of Medicine, Kansas City
1905 University of North Dakota School of Medicine, Grand Forks
1905 University of Utah College of Medicine, Salt Lake City
1907 University of South Dakota School of Medicine, Vermillion
1907 University of Wisconsin Medical School, Madison
1908 Stanford University School of Medicine, Palo Alto
1909 Loma Linda University School of Medicine, Loma Linda
1912 Chicago Medical School University of Health Sciences, Chicago
1913 Medical College of Wisconsin, Milwaukee
1914 Ohio State University College of Medicine, Columbus

1915 Loyola University of Chicago Stritch School of Medicine
1920 University of Rochester School of Medicine and Dentistry, Rochester
1927 University of Chicago Pritzker School of Medicine, Chicago
1930 Duke University School of Medicine, Durham
1931 Louisiana State University School of Medicine, New Orleans
1943 University of Texas Southwestern Medical School, Dallas
1945 University of Washington School of Medicine, Seattle
1949 University of Puerto Rico School of Medicine, San Juan
1951 University of California, School of Medicine, Los Angeles
1952 University of Miami School of Medicine, Miami
1954 University of Kentucky College of Medicine, Lexington
1955 Albert Einstein College of Medicine of Yeshiva University, New York
1956 CMDNJ-New Jersey Medical School, Newark
1956 University of Florida College of Medicine, Gainesville
1960 University of New Mexico School of Medicine, Albuquerque
1962 State University of New York at Stony Brook School of Medicine
1962 University of California College of Medicine, Irvine
1962 University of Massachusetts Medical School, Worcester
1963 Brown University School of Medicine, Providence
1964 Medical College of Ohio at Toledo
1965 University of South Florida College of Medicine, Tampa
1966 Louisiana State University School of Medicine, Shreveport
1966 CMDNJ-Rutgers Medical School, Piscataway
1966 Michigan State University College of Human Medicine, East Lansing
1967 Pennsylvania State University College of Medicine, The Milton S. Hershey Medical Center, Hershey
1967 University of Arizona College of Medicine, Tucson
1967 University of Hawaii School of Medicine, Honolulu
1967 University of Nevada School of Medical Sciences, Reno

1967   University of South Alabama College of Medicine, Mobile
1968   University of California School of Medicine, Davis
1968   University of California School of Medicine, San Diego
1968   University of Missouri School of Medicine, Kansas City
1968   Mount Sinai School of Medicine of the City University of New York
1968   University of Texas Medical School, San Antonio
1968   University of Connecticut School of Medicine, Farmington
1969   Rush Medical College, Chicago
1969   Texas Tech University School of Medicine, Lubbock
1969   University of Texas Medical School, Houston
1969   Southern Illinois University School of Medicine, Springfield
1971   Mayo Medical School, Rochester
1972   University of Minnesota School of Medicine, Duluth
1973   Eastern Virginia Medical School, Norfolk
1973   Wright State University School of Medicine, Dayton

7
Directory Of
Medical Schools

The following listing includes all AMA-accredited medical schools currently accepting applicants. For additional information on the medical schools and on medical school programs, see the following publications:

1975-76 AAMC Curriculum Directory. Washington, D.C.: Association of American Medical Colleges, 1975.

Brown, Sanford J. *Getting Into Medical School*. Woodbury, New York: Barron's Educational Series, Inc., 1975.

Medical School Admission Requirements, 1977-78. Washington, D.C.: Association of American Medical Colleges, 1976.

Wischnitzer, Saul. *Barron's Guide to Medical, Dental, and Allied Health Science Careers*. Woodbury, New York: Barron's Educational Series, Inc., 1977.

How to Read the School Descriptions

The medical schools are listed on the following pages in alphabetical order according to their name, in a strict letter-by-letter arrangement. You will find the complete name of the school and the address to which you should direct any questions or requests for information.

The entries contain the following information: average scores on the MCAT for the first-year class; average grade point average for members of the first-year class; the number of applicants who applied for the most recent class; the percentage who were called for an interview at the school or who were interviewed by alumni at their school or in their hometown; the enrollment of the first-year class; the total enrollment for the medical school; the time during which the school will accept and consider applications; the time during which the school sends out its acceptance notices; and the total average cost of attending the school.

The following abbreviations may be of some additional assistance:

GI	The General Information portion of the Medical College Admission Test
GPA	Grade point average
MCAT	Medical College Admission Test
QA	Quantitative Ability portion of the Medical College Admission Test
Sci	The Science portion of the Medical College Admission Test
VA	Verbal Ability portion of the Medical College Admission Test
WICHE	Western Interstate Commission for Higher Education

Special Note: A new form of the MCAT will be given beginning in May of 1977. This new form of the test will be entirely different from the present examination. The prospective student will be able to use the MCAT scores as given in these entries as a general guide but he or she should be advised that these scores are not comparable with those that will result from the new MCAT.

Albany Medical College of Union University

42 New Scotland Avenue
Albany, NY 12208

MCAT: 622 composite. GPA: 3.5. Number of applicants: 2495 in-state, 1650 out-of-state. Percentage interviewed: 13%. First-year class: 83 men, 27 women; 24% out-of-state. Total enrollment: 335

men, 90 women. Applications: July 1-November 1. Acceptances: December 1-September 15. Total costs: $7385.

Albert Einstein College of Medicine of Yeshiva University
1300 Morris Park Avenue
Bronx, NY 10961

MCAT: Not available. GPA: 3.25. Number of applicants: 2797 in-state, 3450 out-of-state. Percentage interviewed: 27%. First-year class: 130 men, 52 women; 25% out-of-state. Total enrollment: 419 men, 160 women. Applications: July 1-November 1. Acceptances: November 15-(varies). Total costs: $8600.

Baylor College of Medicine
Texas Medical Center
Houston, TX 77030

MCAT: 616 composite. GPA: 3.5. Number of applicants: 1086 in-state, 2346 out-of-state. Percentage interviewed: 22%. First-year class: 133 men, 35 women, 29% out-of-state. Total enrollment: 496 men, 115 women. Applications: June 1 - November 1. Acceptances: November 15 - July 1. Total costs: $3200 instate, $6800 out-of-state.

Boston University School of Medicine
80 East Concord Street
Boston, MA 02118

MCAT: VA-588, QA-633, GI-566, Sci-621. GPA: 3.47. Number of applicants: 4700. Percentage interviewed: 16%. First-year class: 98 men, 41 women; 64% out-of-state. Total enrollment: 394 men, 144 women. Applications: July 1 - November 1. Acceptances: November 15 - (varies). Total costs: $7900.

Bowman Gray School of Medicine of Wake Forest University
300 South Hawthorne Road
Winston-Salem, NC 27103

MCAT: VA-541, QA-601, GI-534, Sci-579. GPA: 3.53. Number of applicants: 474 instate, 3513 out-of-state. Percentage interviewed: 12%. First-year class: 79 men, 22 women, 44% out-of-state. Total enrollment: 305 men, 64 women. Applications: July 1 - November 1. Acceptances: October 1 - September 1. Total costs: $6235.

Brown University Program in Medicine
Providence, RI 02912

MCAT: Not applicable. GPA: Not available. Number of applicants: 38 instate, 87 out-of-state. Percentage interviewed: 25%. First-year class: 43 men, 19 women; 77% out-of-state. Total enrollment: 182 men, 65 women. Applications: August 1 - November 1. Acceptances: November 15 - March 15. Total costs: $6510.

Case Western Reserve University School of Medicine
2119 Abington Road
Cleveland, OH 44106

MCAT: Not available. GPA: Not available. Number of applicants: 1156 instate, 4018 out-of-state. Percentage interviewed: 14%. First-year class: 102 men, 43 women; 40% out-of-state. Total enrollment: 438 men, 143 women. Applications: July 1 - November 15. Acceptances: November 15 - April 15. Total costs: $6295.

College of Medicine and Dentistry of New Jersey
Rutgers Medical School
Box 101
Piscataway, NJ 08854

MCAT: 642 (science). GPA: 3.5. Number of applicants: 1437 instate, 1150 out-of-state. Percentage interviewed: 35%. First-year class: 72 men, 39 women; 17% out-of-state. Total enrollment: 228 men, 99 women. Applications: July 1 - December 15. Acceptances: November 15 - June 1. Total costs: $5350 instate, $6600 out-of-state.

College of Medicine and Dentistry of New Jersey
New Jersey Medical School
100 Bergen Street
Newark, NJ 07103

MCAT: 610 composite. GPA: 3.59. Number of applicants: 1409 instate, 973 out-of-state. Percentage interviewed: 45%. First-year class: 89 men, 30 women; 6% out-of-state. Total enrollment: 376 men, 115 women. Applications: July 1 - December 15. Acceptances: November 15 - date of matriculation. Total costs: $5080 instate, $6330 out-of-state.

Columbia University College of Physicians and Surgeons
630 West 168th Street
New York, NY 10032

MCAT: Not required. GPA: Not available. Number of applicants: 5500 (total). Percentage interviewed: 19%. First-year class: 99 men, 51 women; 40% out-of-state. Total enrollment: 427 men, 175 women. Applications: August 1 - October 15. Acceptances: February 1 - (varies). Total costs: $6375.

Cornell University Medical College
411 East 69th Street
New York, NY 10021

MCAT; 648 (science). GPA: 3.6 (science). Number of applicants: 2978 instate, 5632 out-of-state. Percentage interviewed: 13%. First-year class: 74 men, 28 women; 38% out-of-state. Total enrollment: 317 men, 101 women. Applications: July 1 - November 1. Acceptances: February 1 - March 1. Total costs: $9550.

Creighton University School of Medicine
2500 California Street
Omaha, NE 68178

MCAT: Not available. GPA: 3.40. Number of applicants: 315 instate, 7764 out-of-state. Percentage interviewed: 8%. First-year class: 99 men, 11 women; 75% out-of-state. Total enrollment: 392 men, 47 women. Applications: July 1 - December 15. Acceptances: January 1 - date of matriculation. Total costs: $6725.

Dartmouth Medical School
Hanover, NH 03755

MCAT: Not available. GPA: Not available. Number of applicants: 68 instate, 2900 out-of-state. Percentage interviewed: 10%. First-year class: 51 men, 17 women; 88% out-of-state. Total enrollment: 125 men, 41 women. Applications: June 1 - November 1. Acceptances: November 15 - August 1. Total costs: $8210.

Duke University School of Medicine
Box 3710
Durham, NC 27710

MCAT: Not available. GPA: Not available. Number of applicants: 316 instate, 3808 out-of-state. Percentage interviewed: 54%. First-year class: 84 men, 35 women; 70% out-of-state. Total enrollment: 372 men, 113 women. Applications: August 1 - November 1. Acceptances: November - March. Total costs: $6475.

Eastern Virginia Medical School
358 Mowbray Arch, Box 1980
Norfolk, VA 23501

MCAT: 585 composite. GPA: 3.25. Number of applicants: 575 instate, 850 out-of-state. Percentage interviewed: 17%. First-year class: 34 men, 14 women; 12% out-of-state. Total enrollment: 81 men, 26 women. Applications: July 1 - December 1. Acceptances: December 15 - July 1. Total costs: $7675 instate, $8675 out-of-state.

Emory University School of Medicine
Atlanta, GA 30322

MCAT: VA-590, QA-635, GI-565, Sci-625. GPA: 3.48. Number of applicants: 403 instate, 4216 out-of-state. Percentage interviewed: 13*. First-year class: 81 men, 31 women; 48* out-of-state. Total enrollment: 368 men, 74 women. Applications: July 1-October 15. Acceptances: December 1-March 31. Total costs: $6600.

Georgetown University School of Medicine
3900 Reservoir Road, N.W.
Washington, DC 20007

MCAT: VA-604, QA-636, GI-580, Sci-647. GPA: 3.48. Number of applicants: 111 resident, 9089 nonresident. Percentage interviewed: 16%. First-year class: 168 men, 42 women; 94% nonresident. Total enrollment: 672 men, 145 women. Applications: July 1 - November 1. Acceptances: November 15- August. Total cost: Not available.

George Washington University
School of Medicine and Health Sciences
2300 Eye Street, N.W.
Washington, DC 20037

MCAT: 607 composite. GPA: 3.3. Number of applicants: 122 resident, 9502 nonresident. Percentage interviewed: 8%. First-year class: 108 men, 44 women; 92% nonresident. Total enrollment: 459 men, 143 women. Applications: July 1 - November 15. Acceptances: November 15- Summer. Total costs: Not available.

Hahnemann Medical College
245 North 15th Street
Philadelphia, PA 19102

MCAT: Not available. GPA: 3.4. Number of applicants: 2087 instate, 3117 out-of-state. Percentage interviewed: 19%. First-year class: 145

men, 37 women; 23% out-of-state. Total enrollment: 551 men, 121 women. Applications: July 1 - November 15. Acceptances: September 1 - September 15. Total costs: $8650.

Harvard Medical School
25 Shattuck Street
Boston, MA 02115

MCAT: Not available. GPA: Not available. Number of applicants: 293 instate, 2825 out-of-state. Percentage interviewed: 38%. First-year class: 106 men, 59 women; 90% out-of-state. Total enrollment: 468 men, 196 women. Applications: June - November 1. Acceptances: December 1 - February 18. Total costs: $7650.

Howard University College of Medicine
520 W Street, N.W.
Washington, DC 20059

MCAT: Not available. GPA: Not available. Number of applicants: 194 resident, 3899 nonresident. Percentage interviewed: 10%. First-year class: 90 men, 44 women; 90% nonresident. Total enrollment: 328 men, 146 women. Applications: July 1 - December 15. Acceptances: December 1 - (varies). Total costs: $6100.

Indiana University School of Medicine
1100 W. Michigan Street
Indianapolis, IN 46201

MCAT: Not available. GPA: Not available. Number of applicants: 817 instate, 958 out-of-state. Percentage interviewed: 60%. First-year class: 264 men, 54 women; 1% out-of-state. Total enrollment: 1010 men, 196 women. Applications: July 1 - December 15. Acceptances: December 15 - June 30. Total costs: $4150 instate, $6300 out-of-state.

Jefferson Medical College of Thomas Jefferson University
1025 Walnut Street
Philadelphia, PA 19107

MCAT: QA-635, Sci-644. GPA: 3.52 (science), 3.49 (nonscience). Number of applicants: 2092 instate, 3182 out-of-state. Percentage interviewed: 16%. First-year class: 182 men, 47 women; 27% out-of-state. Total enrollment: 739 men, 154 women. Applications: July 1 - November 15. Acceptances: November 15 - June 1. Total costs: $7452.

Johns Hopkins University School of Medicine
725 North Wolfe Street
Baltimore, MD 21205

MCAT: Not available. GPA: Not available. Number of applicants: 190 instate, 2624 out-of-state. Percentage interviewed: 32%. First-year class: 99 men, 23 women; 88% out-of-state. Total enrollment: 393 men, 87 women. Applications: June 1 - October 15. Acceptances: November 15 - March 15. Total costs: $6350.

Loma Linda University School of Medicine
Loma Linda, CA 92354

MCAT: Not available. GPA: Not available. Number of applicants: 1581 instate, 3145 out-of-state. Percentage interviewed: 20%. First-year class: 123 men, 39 women; 67% out-of-state. Total enrollment: 467 men, 106 women. Applications: July 1 - November 1. Acceptances: February 15 - April. Total costs: $8520.

Louisiana State University Medical Center
School of Medicine in New Orleans
1542 Tulane Avenue
New Orleans, LA 70112

MCAT: QA-577, Sci-575. GPA: 3.41. Number of applicants: 741 instate, 373 out-of-state. Percentage interviewed: 65%. First-year class: 143 men, 39 women; 0% out-of-state. Total enrollment: 508 men, 104 women. Applications: July 1 - November 15. Acceptances: December 15 - (varies). Total costs: $3900.

Louisiana State University Medical Center
School of Medicine in Shreveport
Box 3932
Shreveport, LA 71130

MCAT: QA-590, Sci-590. GPA: 3.6. Number of applicants: 518 instate, 199 out-of-state. Percentage interviewed: 33%. First-year class: 83 men, 16 women; 0% out-of-state. Total enrollment: 205 men, 24 women. Applications: July 1 - November 15. Acceptances: December 15 - February 15. Total costs: $3250 instate, $4750 out-of-state.

Loyola University of Chicago
Stritch School of Medicine
2160 South First Avenue
Maywood, IL 60153

MCAT: Not available. GPA: Not available. Number of applicants: 1550 instate, 4280 out-of-state. Percentage interviewed: 6%. First-year class: 100 men, 35 women; 28% out-of-state. Total enrollment: 316 men, 88 women. Applications: July - November 15. Acceptances: September - until class is enrolled. Total costs: $9100.

Mayo Medical School
200 First Street, S.W.
Rochester, MN 55901

MCAT: 603 composite. GPA: 3.61. Number of applicants: 732 instate, 860 out-of-state. Percentage interviewed: 46% instate, 2%

out-of-state. First-year class: 30 men, 10 women; 12% out-of-state. Total enrollment: 127 men, 32 women. Applications: July 1 - November 15. Acceptances: December 15 - May 15. Total costs: $5450 instate, $6550 out-of-state.

Medical College of Georgia School of Medicine
Augusta, GA 30902

MCAT: 570 composite. GPA: 3.4. Number of applicants: 621 instate, 761 out-of-state. Percentage interviewed: 32%. First-year class: 140 men, 4% out-of-state. Total enrollment: 572 men, 113 women. Applications: July 1 - December 1. Acceptances: December 15 - date of matriculation. Total costs: $3500 instate, $4700 out-of-state.

Medical College of Ohio
Box 6190
Toledo, OH 43614

MCAT: VA-545, QA-603, GI-540, Sci-594. GPA: 3.54. Number of applicants: 1409 instate, 513 out-of-state. Percentage interviewed: 25%. First-year class: 72 men, 27 women; 4% out-of-state. Total enrollment: 189 men, 59 women. Applications: July 1 - November 15. Acceptances: December 15 - June. Total costs: $2400 instate, $3200 out-of-state, exclusive of room & board.

Medical College of Pennsylvania
3300 Henry Avenue
Philadelphia, PA 19129

MCAT: VA-586, QA-622, GI-555, Sci-606. GPA: 3.45. Number of applicants: 1936 instate, 2760 out-of-state. Percentage interviewed: 12%. First-year class: 37 men, 67 women; 21.5% out-of-state. Total enrollment: 132 men, 256 women. Applications: July 1 - December 1. Acceptances: September 1 - June 15. Total costs: $8200.

Medical College of Virginia School of Medicine
Box 636, MCV Station
Richmond, VA 23298

MCAT: 577 composite. GPA: 3.43. Number of applicants: 776 instate, 2576 out-of-state. Percentage interviewed: 22%. First-year class: 132 men, 37 women; 9% out-of-state. Total enrollment: 501 men, 105 women. Applications: July 1 - December 1. Acceptances: November 15 - until class is enrolled. Total costs: $4145 instate, $5665 out-of-state.

Medical College of Wisconsin
561 North 15th Street
Milwaukee, WI 53233

MCAT: VA-575 resident (605 nonresident), QA-645 (665), GI-545 (575), Sci-645 (695). GPA: 3.63 resident (3.70 nonresident). Number of applicants: 568 instate, 3162 out-of-state. Percentage interviewed: 10%. First-year class: 100 men, 25 women; 33% out-of-state. Total enrollment: 422 men, 74 women. Applications: July 1 - December 1. Acceptances: November 15 - August 26. Total costs: $5800 instate, $6800 out-of-state.

Medical University of South Carolina
College of Medicine
80 Barre Street
Charleston, SC 24901

MCAT: Not available. GPA: Not available. Number of applicants: 494 instate, 774 out-of-state. Percentage interviewed: 31%. First-year class: 147 men, 28 women; 2% out-of-state. Total enrollment: 570 men, 88 women. Applications: July 1 - December 1. Acceptances: October 1 - March 1. Total costs: $3075 instate, $3915 out-of-state.

Meharry Medical College School of Medicine
1005 18th Avenue, North
Nashville, TN 37208

MCAT: Not available. GPA: Not available. Number of applicants: 385 instate, 2798 out-of-state. Percentage interviewed: 6%. First-year class: 94 men, 32 women; 85% out-of-state. Total enrollment: 316 men, 117 women. Applications: March 15 - January 2. Acceptances: November 15 - May 30. Total costs: $4780.

Michigan State University College of Human Medicine
A234 Life Sciences Building
East Lansing, MI 48824

MCAT: Not available. GPA: Not available. Number of applicants: 1800 instate, 1000 out-of-state. Percentage interviewed: 10%. First-year class: 65 men, 40 women; 20% out-of-state. Total enrollment: 257 men, 146 women. Applications: July 1 - December 1. Acceptances: December 15 - (varies). Total costs: $3825 instate, $5175 out-of-state.

Mount Sinai School of Medicine of the
City University of New York
Fifth Avenue and 100th Street
New York, NY 10029

MCAT: 606 composite. GPA: 3.5. Number of applicants: 2386 instate, 1512 out-of-state. Percentage interviewed: 20%. First-year class: 67 men, 18 women; 24% out-of-state. Total enrollment: 255 men, 78 women. Applications: August 1 - October 31. Acceptances: November 15 - (varies). Total costs: $7780.

New York Medical College
Elmwood Hall
Valhalla, NY 10595

MCAT: 605 composite. GPA: 3.63. Number of applicants: 2939 instate, 1966 out-of-state. Percentage interviewed: 18%. First-year class: 123 men, 57 women; 30% out-of-state. Total enrollment: 567 men, 164 women. Applications: July 1 - November 15. Acceptances: November 15 - July. Total costs: $7568.

New York University School of Medicine
550 First Avenue
New York, NY 10016

MCAT: Not available. GPA: Not available. Number of applicants: 4631 (total). Percentage interviewed: 43%. First-year class: 120 men, 51 women; 29% out-of-state. Total enrollment: 530 men, 163 women. Applications: September 1 - December 31. Acceptances: December 15 - (varies). Total costs: $7305.

Northwestern University Medical School
303 East Chicago Avenue
Chicago, IL 60611

MCAT: VA-596, QA-648, GI-564, Sci-650. GPA: 3.54. Number of applicants: 1307 instate, 5292 out-of-state. Percentage interviewed: 22%. First-year class: 128 men, 42 women; 50% out-of-state. Total enrollment: 545 men, 153 women. Applications: July 1 - November 15. Acceptances: February 1 - (varies). Total costs: $7900.

Ohio State University College of Medicine
370 West Ninth Avenue
Columbus, OH 43210

MCAT: Not available. GPA: 3.6. Number of applicants: 1518 instate, 771 out-of-state. Percentage interviewed: 35%. First-year class: 198 men, 45 women; 1% out-of-state. Total enrollment: 596 men, 123 women. Applications: July 1 - December 15. Acceptances: October 15 - until class is enrolled. Total costs: $4955 instate, $6355 out-of-state.

Pennsylvania State University College of Medicine
Milton S. Hershey Medical Center
Hershey PA 17033

MCAT: 600 composite. GPA: 3.6. Number of applicants: 1595 instate, 965 out-of-state. Percentage interviewed: 20%. First-year class: 78 men, 23 women; 10% out-of-state. Total enrollment: 282 men, 74 women. Applications: July 1 - December 1. Acceptances: September 15 - until class is enrolled. Total costs: $5264 instate, $7265 out-of-state.

Rush Medical College of Rush University
1743 West Harrison Street
Chicago, IL 60612

MCAT: Not available. GPA: Not available. Number of applicants: 1412 instate, 1974 out-of-state. Percentage interviewed: 17%. First-year class: 80 men, 32 women; 5% out-of-state. Total enrollment: 251 men, 83 women. Applications: July 1 - November 15. Acceptances: December 15 - date of matriculation. Total costs: $7800.

Saint Louis University School of Medicine
1402 South Grand Boulevard
St. Louis, MO 63104

MCAT: QA-641, Sci-639. GPA: 3.61. Number of applicants: 516 instate, 8414 out-of-state. Percentage interviewed: 16%. First-year class: 131 men, 23 women; 64% out-of-state. Total enrollment: 512 men, 84 women. Applications: July 1 - December 15. Acceptances: November 15 - August 28. Total costs: $5778.

Southern Illinois University School of Medicine
Box 3926
Springfield, IL 62708

MCAT: VA-544, QA-606, GI-523, Sci-617. GPA: 3.33. Number of applicants: 1100 instate, 142 out-of-state. Percentage interviewed: 50%. First-year class: 60 men, 10 women; 0% out-of-state. Total enrollment: 143 men, 23 women. Applications: July 1 - November 15. Acceptances: November 15 - February 15. Total costs: $4140 instate, $5430 out-of-state.

Stanford University School of Medicine
851 Welch Road, Room 154
Palo Alto, CA 94304

MCAT: Not available. GPA: 3.5. Number of applicants: Not available. Percentage interviewed: 16%. First-year class: 60 men, 26 women: 52% out-of-state. Total enrollment: 292 men, 106 women. Applications: July 1-November 1. Acceptances: December 15-March 15. Total costs: $8500.

State University of New York at Buffalo
School of Medicine
Farber Hall, Room 135
Buffalo, NY 14214

MCAT: Not available. GPA: 3.4. Number of applicants: 3695 instate, 921 out-of-state. Percentage interviewed: 12%. First-year class: 96 men, 48 women; 5% out-of-state. Total enrollment: 420 men, 136 women. Applications: July 1-December 15. Acceptances: November 15-August. Total costs: $4200 instate, $4600 out-of-state.

State University of New York at Stony Brook
Health Sciences Center / School of Medicine
Stony Brook, NY 11794

MCAT: not available. GPA: Not available. Number of applicants: 2600 (total). Percentage interviewed: 19%. First-year class: 26 men,

23 women; 10% out-of-state. Total enrollment: 72 men, 63 women. Applications: July 1 - December 15. Acceptances: November - March. Total costs: $4750 instate, $5150 out-of-state.

State University of New York/Downstate Medical Center School of Medicine
450 Clarkson Avenue
Brooklyn, NY 14214

MCAT: 612 composite. GPA: 3.5. Number of applicants: 3821 instate, 1266 out-of-state. Percentage interviewed: 20%. First-year class: 165 men, 59 women; 5% out-of-state. Total enrollment: 702 men, 184 women. Applications: July 1 - December 15. Acceptances: November 15 - September 1. Total costs: $5700 instate, $6700 out-of-state.

State University of New York Upstate Medical Center College of Medicine
155 Elizabeth Blackwell Street
Syracuse, NY 13210

MCAT: QA-643, Sci-651. GPA: 3.47. Number of applicants: 3735 instate, 662 out-of-state. Percentage interviewed: 15%. First-year class: 88 men, 36% women; 0% out-of-state. Total enrollment: 380 men, 106 women. Applications: July 1 - December 15. Acceptances: November 15 - April 1. Total costs: $3955 instate, $4355 out-of-state.

Temple University School of Medicine
Broad & Tioga Streets
Philadelphia, PA 19140

MCAT: QA-589, Sci-576. GPA: 3.26. Number of applicants: 2332 instate, 2467 out-of-state. Percentage interviewed: 22%. First-year class: 148 men, 38 women; 10% out-of-state. Total enrollment: 578 men, 147 women. Applications: July 1 - December 1. Acceptances: October - June. Total costs: $4575 instate, $6575 out-of-state.

Texas Tech University School of Medicine
Box 4569
Lubbock, TX 79409

MCAT: 588 composite. GPA: 3.35. Number of applicants: 1004 instate, 326 out-of-state. Percentage interviewed: 20%. First-year class: 38 men, 6 women; 0% out-of-state. Total enrollment: 105 men, 27 women. Applications: July 1 - November 1. Acceptances: January 15 - May. Total costs: $4125 instate, $4658 out-of-state.

Tufts University School of Medicine
136 Harrison Avenue
Boston, MA 02111

MCAT: Not available. GPA: Not available. Number of applicants: 713 instate, 7033 out-of-state. Percentage interviewed: 10%. First-year class: 99 men, 51 women; 71% out-of-state. Total enrollment: 437 men, 180 women. Applications: July 1 - November 1. Acceptances: December 15 - (varies). Total costs: $8100.

Tulane University School of Medicine
1403 Tulane Avenue
New Orleans, LA 70112

MCAT: Not available. GPA: Not available. Number of applicants: 481 instate, 4904 out-of-state. Percentage interviewed: 15%. First-year class: 116 men, 33 women; 51% out-of-state. Total enrollment: 490 men, 104 women. Applications: July 1 - December 15. Acceptances: December 15 - (varies). Total costs: $5930 instate, $6430 out-of-state.

University of Alabama School of Medicine
University Station
Birmingham, AL 35294

MCAT: 555 composite. GPA: 3.47. Number of applicants: 487 in-state, 497 out-of-state. Percentage interviewed: 49%. First-year class: 113 men, 32 women; 2% out-of-state. Total enrollment: 331 men, 73 women. Applications: July 1 - November 1. Acceptances: January 15 - date of matriculation. Total costs: $6100 instate, $7700 out-of-state.

University of Arizona College of Medicine
Tucson, AZ 85724

MCAT: 610 composite. GPA: 3.6. Number of applicants: 390 instate, 310 out-of-state. Percentage interviewed: 54%. First-year class: 61 men, 38 women; 0% out-of-state. Total enrollment: 196 men, 78 women. Applications: July 1 - November 1. Acceptances: January 15 - until class is enrolled. Total costs: $4050 instate, $5240 out-of-state.

University of Arkansas College of Medicine
4301 West Markham Street
Little Rock, AR 72201

MCAT: 580 composite. GPA: 3.5. Number of applicants: 324 instate, 323 out-of-state. Percentage interviewed: 100% instate. First-year class: 93 men, 30 women; 0% out-of-state. Total enrollment: 411 men, 71 women. Applications: July 1 - November 15. Acceptances: December 15 - (varies). Total costs: $3670 instate, $4040 out-of-state.

University of California, Davis
School of Medicine
Davis, CA 95616

MCAT: Not available. GPA: Not available. Number of applicants: 3209 instate, 437 out-of-state. Percentage interviewed: 13%. First-year class: 73 men, 29 women; 1% out-of-state. Total enrollment: 296 men, 114 women. Applications: July 1 - November 1. Acceptances: December 15 - (varies). Total costs: $3270 instate, $4770 out-of-state.

University of California, Irvine
California College of Medicine
Irvine, CA 92717

MCAT: Not available. GPA: Not available. Number of applicants: 2939 instate, 574 out-of-state. Percentage interviewed: 28%. First-year class: 65 men, 14 women; 1.4% out-of-state. Total enrollment: 248 men, 61 women. Applications: July 1 - November 15. Acceptances: November 15 - June 30. Total costs: $5200 instate, $6700 out-of-state.

University of California, Los Angeles
School of Medicine
Center for Health and Sciences
Los Angeles, CA 90024

MCAT: 618 composite. GPA: 3.54. Number of applicants: 2697 instate, 1068 out-of-state. Percentage interviewed: 20%. First-year class: 107 men, 39 women; 7% out-of-state. Total enrollment: 512 men, 110 women. Applications: July 1 - November 1. Acceptances: January 15 - September. Total costs: $4500 instate, $6000 out-of-state.

University of California, San Diego
School of Medicine
Box 109
La Jolla, CA 92093

MCAT: 640 composite. GPA: 3.6. Number of applicants: 2651 in-state, 1439 out-of-state. Percentage interviewed: 11%. First-year class: 84 men, 12 women; 12% out-of-state. Total enrollment: 264 men, 56 women. Applications: July 1 - November 1. Acceptances: December 15 - (varies). Total costs: $5100 instate, $6600 out-of-state.

University of California, San Francisco
School of Medicine
San Francisco, CA 94143

MCAT: 645 composite. GPA: 3.5. Number of applicants: 2768 in-state, 1804 out-of-state. Percentage interviewed: 20%. First-year class: 91 men, 57 women; 16% out-of-state. Total enrollment: 424 men, 189 women. Applications: July 1 - November 1. Acceptances: January 15 - until class is enrolled. Total costs: $3100 instate, $4600 out-of-state.

University of Chicago
Pritzker School of Medicine
5724 South Ellis Avenue
Chicago, IL 60637

MCAT: 635 composite. GPA: 3.68 science, 3.63 nonscience. Number of applicants: 810 instate, 4534 out-of-state. Percentage interviewed: 7%. First-year class: 85 men, 19 women; 60% out-of-state. Total enrollment: 372 men, 77 women. Applications: July 1 - December 1. Acceptances: November 15 - April 15. Total costs: $6200.

University of Cincinnati School of Medicine
231 Bethesda Avenue
Cincinnati, OH 45267

MCAT: 587 composite. GPA: 3.41. Number of applicants: 1427 instate, 4346 out-of-state. Percentage interviewed: 21%. First-year class: 150 men, 44 women; 25% out-of-state. Total enrollment: 521 men, 115 women. Applications: July 1 - December 15. Acceptances: December 15 - September 1. Total costs: $3800 city resident, $3950 state resident, $5300 out-of-state.

University of Colorado School of Medicine
4200 East Ninth Avenue
Denver, CO 80220

MCAT: QA-635, VA-597, GI-554, Sci-635. GPA: 3.57. Number of applicants: 485 instate, 1156 out-of-state. Percentage interviewed: 31%. First-year class: 97 men, 31 women; 18% out-of-state. Total enrollment: 407 men, 119 women. Applications: July 1 - November 1. Acceptances: December 15 - March 15. Total costs: $3900 instate, $7900 out-of-state.

University of Connecticut School of Medicine
The University of Connecticut Health Center
School of Medicine
Farmington, CT 06032

MCAT: VA-612, QA-640, GI-592, Sci-641. GPA: 3.49. Number of applicants: 574 instate, 1142 out-of-state. Percentage interviewed: 17%. First-year class: 56 men, 24 women; 12% out-of-state. Total enrollment: 210 men, 62 women. Applications: July 1 - December 1. Acceptances: November 15 - September 1. Total costs: 3750 instate, $4650 out-of-state.

University of Florida College of Medicine
J. Hillis Miller Health Center
Gainesville, FL 32610

MCAT: 600 composite. GPA: 3.5. Number of applicants: 919 instate, 1198 out-of-state. Percentage interviewed: 16%. First-year class: 95 men, 25 women; 10% out-of-state. Total enrollment: 348 men, 85 women. Applications: July 1 - December 15. Acceptances: October 15 - until class is enrolled. Total costs: $3645 instate, $4950 out-of-state.

University of Hawaii
John A. Burns School of Medicine
1960 East-West Road
Honolulu, HI 96822

MCAT: Not available. GPA: Not available. Number of applicants: 228 instate, 2688 out-of-state. Percentage interviewed: 10%. First-year class: 45 men, 21 women; 7% out-of-state. Total enrollment: 206 men, 58 women. Applications: July 1 - December 15. Acceptances: December 15 - March 15. Total costs: $5550 instate, $8550 out-of-state.

University of Health Sciences
The Chicago Medical School
2020 West Ogden Avenue
Chicago, IL 60612

MCAT: 585 composite. GPA: 3.49. Number of applicants: 1194 instate, 5784 out-of-state. Percentage interviewed: 8%. First-year class: 82 men, 33 women; 40% out-of-state. Total enrollment: 336 men, 54 women. Applications: July 1 - December 15. Acceptances: November 15 - June 1. Total costs: $7650.

University of Illinois College of Medicine
1737 West Polk Street
Chicago, IL 60612

MCAT: Not available. GPA: Not available. Number of applicants: 1781 instate, 755 out-of-state. Percentage interviewed: 10%. First-year class: 270 men, 79 women; .3% out-of-state. Total enrollment: 1047 men, 222 women. Applications: July 1 - December 15. Acceptances: November 15 - March 30. Total costs: $4200 instate, $5200 out-of-state.

University of Iowa College of Medicine
Iowa City, IA 52242

MCAT: Not available. GPA: Not available. Number of applicants: 429 instate, 509 out-of-state. Percentage interviewed: 1%. First-year class: 143 men, 32 women; 5% out-of-state. Total enrollment: 561 men, 112 women. Applications: July 1 - December 1. Acceptances: December 15 - August. Total costs: $3400 instate, $4850 out-of-state.

University of Kansas School of Medicine
39th Street and Rainbow Boulevard
Kansas City, KS 66103

MCAT: 580 composite. GPA: Not available. Number of applicants: 461 instate, 628 out-of-state. Percentage interviewed: 45%. First-year class: 187 men, 29 women, 6.5% out-of-state. Total enrollment: 476 men, 89 women. Applications: April 1 - November 15. Acceptances: January 15 - August. Total costs: $5200 instate, $6700 out-of-state.

University of Kentucky College of Medicine
800 Rose Street
Lexington, KY 40506

MCAT: 574 composite. GPA: 3.4. Number of applicants: 512 instate, 1106 out-of-state. Percentage interviewed: 20%. First-year class: 87 men, 26 women; 6.5% out-of-state. Total enrollment: 345 men, 85 women. Applications: July 1-November 15. Acceptances: November 15-September 1. Total costs: $2600 instate, $3500 out-of-state.

University of Louisville School of Medicine
Health Sciences Center
Louisville, KY 40201

MCAT: 565 composite. GPA: 3.60. Number of applicants: 501 instate, 743 out-of-state. Percentage interviewed: 22%. First-year class: 107 men, 31 women; 12% out-of-state. Total enrollment: 442 men, 101 women. Applications: July 1 - December 15. Acceptances: November 15 - until class is enrolled. Total costs: $3700 instate, $4700 out-of-state.

University of Maryland School of Medicine
660 West Redwood Street
Baltimore, MD 21201

MCAT: VA-584, QA-641, GI-565, Sci-625. GPA: 3.57. Number of applicants: 821 instate, 821 out-of-state. Percentage interviewed: 30%. First-year class: 126 men, 41 women; 8% out-of-state. Total enrollment: 514 men, 121 women. Applications: July 1 - December 1. Acceptances: November 15 - April 15. Total costs: $5100 instate, $6600 out-of-state.

University of Massachusetts Medical School
55 Lake Avenue, North
Worcester, MA 01605

MCAT: Not available. GPA: 3.25 (science). Number of applicants: 986 instate. Percentage interviewed: 20%. First-year class: 76 men, 26 women; 0% out-of-state. Total enrollment: 177 men, 55 women. Applications: July 1 - December 15. Acceptances: December 15 - date of matriculation. Total costs: $2970.

University of Miami School of Medicine

Box 520875, Biscayne Annex
Miami, FL 33152

MCAT: Not available. GPA: Not available. Number of applicants: 1306 instate, 585 out-of-state. Percentage interviewed: 100%. First-year class: 136 men, 26 women; 3% out-of-state. Total enrollment: 511 men, 76 women. Applications: July 1 - December 15. Acceptances: October 15 - March 1. Total costs: $6700.

University of Michigan Medical School

1335 Catherine Street
Ann Arbor, MI 48104

MCAT: 607 composite. GPA: 3.62. Number of applicants: 1537 instate, 2492 out-of-state. Percentage interviewed: 24%. First-year class: 175 men, 72 women; 18% out-of-state. Total enrollment: 721 men, 225 women. Applications: July 1 - December 15. Acceptances: (Varies) - September 1. Total costs: $6200 instate, $8200 out-of-state.

University of Minnesota Duluth School of Medicine

2205 East Fifth Street
Duluth, MN 55812

MCAT: QA-619, Sci-601. GPA: 3.44. Number of applicants: 704 instate, 172 out-of-state. Percentage interviewed: 33%. First-year class: 32 men, 4 women; 14% out-of-state. Total enrollment: 61 men, 12 women. Applications: July 1 - November 15. Acceptances: December 15 - (varies). Total costs: $4700 instate, $8000 out-of-state.

University of Minnesota Medical School Minneapolis

Box 282, Mayo Memorial Building
Minneapolis, MN 55455

MCAT: 600 composite. GPA: 3.44. Number of applicants: 896 instate, 1152 out-of-state. Percentage interviewed: 30%. First-year class: 199 men, 49 women; 4% out-of-state. Total enrollment: 818 men, 178 women. Applications: July 1 - November 15. Acceptances: December 15 - May 15. Total costs: $5815 instate, $9115 out-of-state.

University of Mississippi School of Medicine
2500 North State Street
Jackson, MS 39216

MCAT: 550 composite. GPA: 3.4. Number of applicants: 355 instate, 340 out-of-state. Percentage interviewed: 35%. First-year class: 122 men, 29 women; 0% out-of-state. Total enrollment: 451 men, 79 women. Applications: July 1 - December 1. Acceptances: November 15 - (varies). Total costs: $3875 instate, $4575 out-of-state.

University of Missouri/Columbia
School of Medicine
Columbia, MO 65201

MCAT: Not available. GPA: Not available. Number of applicants: 636 instate, 865 out-of-state. Percentage interviewed: 70%. First-year class: 88 men, 28 women; 0% out-of-state. Total enrollment: 367 men, 81 women. Applications: July 1 - November 15. Acceptances: November 1 - (varies). Total costs: $2375.

University of Missouri/Kansas City
School of Medicine
5100 Rockhill Road
Kansas City, MO 64110

MCAT: Not available. GPA: Not available. Number of applicants: 455 instate. Percentage interviewed: 86%. First-year class: 39 men, 23 women; 0% out-of-state. Total enrollment: 141 men, 58 women. Applications: July 1 - January 1. Acceptances: March 1 - May 1. Total costs: $2215 (Years 1 & 2), $3300 (Years 3-6) instate; $3565 (Years 1 & 2), $4970 (Years 3-6), out-of-state.

University of Nebraska College of Medicine
42nd Street and Dewey Avenue
Omaha, NE 68105

MCAT: 559 composite. GPA: 3.52. Number of applicants: 500 instate, 623 out-of-state. Percentage interviewed: 45%. First-year class: 130 men, 25 women; 7% out-of-state. Total enrollment: 395 men, 69 women. Applications: July 1 - November 15. Acceptances: December 15 - April 15. Total costs: $5000 instate, $6050 out-of-state.

University of Nevada School of Medicine
Reno, NV 89507

MCAT: 580 overall, 610 science. GPA: 3.4. Number of applicants: 120 instate, 525 out-of-state. Percentage interviewed: 30%. First-year class: 39 men, 9 women; 10% out-of-state. Total enrollment: 77 men, 20 women. Applications: July 1 - December 1. Acceptances: December 15 - summer. Total costs: $5750 instate, $9950 out-of-state.

University of New Mexico School of Medicine
Health Sciences Center
Albuquerque, NM 87131

MCAT: 573 composite. GPA: 3.35. Number of applicants: 278 instate, 858 out-of-state. Percentage interviewed: 30%. First-year class: 62 men, 16 women; 14% out-of-state. Total enrollment: 212 men, 70 women. Applications: July 1 - December 15. Acceptances: December 15 - March 15. Total costs: $3000 instate, $3875 out-of-state.

University of North Carolina School of Medicine
Chapel Hill, NC 27514

MCAT: Not available. GPA: 3.44. Number of applicants: 630 instate, 1044 out-of-state. Percentage interviewed: 33%. First-year class: 109 men, 31 women; 7% out-of-state. Total enrollment: 413 men, 110 women. Applications: July 1 - December 15. Acceptances: November 15 - date of matriculation. Total costs: $3365 instate, $5120 out-of-state.

University of North Dakota School of Medicine
Grand Forks, ND 58202

MCAT: Not available. GPA: Not available. Number of applicants: 168 instate, 40 out-of-state. Percentage interviewed: 100% (instate). First-year class: 56 men, 12 women: 7% out-of-state. Total enrollment: 186 men, 27 women. Applications: August 1 - November 1. Acceptances: December 15 - August 15. Total costs: $2600 instate, $3450 out-of-state.

University of Oklahoma College of Medicine
Box 26901
Oklahoma City, OK 73190

MCAT: 568 composite. GPA: 3.55. Number of applicants: 480 instate, 737 out-of-state. Percentage interviewed: 35%. First-year class: 145 men, 23 women; 5% out-of-state. Total enrollment: 536 men, 82 women. Applications: July 1 - November 1. Acceptances: (Varies) - April 15. Total costs: $5125 instate, $6045 out-of-state.

University of Oregon Health Sciences Center
School of Medicine
3181 S.W. Sam Jackson Park Road
Portland, OR 97201

MCAT: VA-585, QA-645, GI-555, Sci-645. GPA: 3.6. Number of applicants: 383 instate, 188 WICHE, 275 other out-of-state. Percentage interviewed: 100% instate, 10% WICHE, 2% other out-of-state. First-year class: 91 men, 24 women; 5% out-of-state. Total enrollment: 382 men, 79 women. Applications: July 1 - November 15.

Acceptances: December 15 - March 15. Total costs: $4600 instate, $6000 out-of-state.

University of Pennsylvania School of Medicine
36th & Hamilton Walk
Philadelphia, PA 19174

MCAT: Not available. GPA: Not available. Number of applicants: 1496 instate, 3321 out-of-state. Percentage interviewed: 20%. First-year class: 116 men, 44 women; 43% out-of-state. Total enrollment: 498 men, 150 women. Applications: July 1 - November 1. Acceptances: December 1 - March. Total costs: $7600.

University of Pittsburgh School of Medicine
3550 Terrace Street
Pittsburgh, PA 15261

MCAT: 613 composite. GPA: 3.54. Number of applicants: 1854 instate, 1975 out-of-state. Percentage interviewed: 19%. First-year class: 102 men, 35 women; 14% out-of-state. Total enrollment: 418 men, 117 women. Applications: July 1 - November 15. Acceptances: September 15 - (varies). Total costs: $5700 instate, $7700 out-of-state.

University of Puerto Rico School of Medicine
Medical Sciences Campus, Box 5067
San Juan, PR 00936

MCAT: 1973 (total). GPA: 3.5. Number of applicants: 459 resident, 92 nonresident. Percentage interviewed: 64%. First-year class: 89 men, 46 women; no nonresidents. Total enrollment: 338 men, 137 women. Applications: July 1 - December 15. Acceptances: March 15 - (varies). Total costs: $2420.

University of Rochester School of Medicine and Dentistry
Box 601
Rochester, NY 14642

MCAT: Not available. GPA: 3.6. Number of applicants: 4523 (total). Percentage interviewed: 15%. First-year class: 72 men, 26 women; 45% out-of-state. Total enrollment: 311 men, 80 women. Applications: August - November 15. Acceptances: November 15 - May 15. Total costs: $7265.

University of South Alabama College of Medicine
Mobile, AL 36688

MCAT: Not available. GPA: Not available. Number of applicants: 452 instate, 561 out-of-state. Percentage interviewed: 45%. First-year class: 58 men, 8 women; 0% out-of-state. Total enrollment: 179 men, 34 women. Applications: July 1 - November 1. Acceptances: January 15 - March 15. Total costs: $3800.

University of South Dakota School of Medicine
Vermillion, SD 57069

MCAT: VA-560, QA-596, GI-529, Sci-577. GPA: 3.43 (science), 3.44 (nonscience). Number of applicants: 119 instate, 493 out-of-state. Percentage interviewed: 20%. First-year class: 51 men, 14 women; 1.5% out-of-state. Total enrollment: 139 men, 29 women. Applications: July 1 - December 15. Acceptances: December 15 - (varies). Total costs: $2800 instate, $4130 out-of-state.

University of Southern California School of Medicine
2025 Zonal Avenue
Los Angeles, CA 90033

MCAT: Not available. GPA: Not available. Number of applicants: 2560 instate, 1622 out-of-state. Percentage interviewed: 23%. First-year class: 119 men, 20 women; 18% out-of-state. Total enrollment: 417 men, 99 women. Applications: July - November 1. Acceptances: November 15 - until class is enrolled. Total costs: $7100.

University of South Florida College of Medicine
Tampa, FL 33620

MCAT: Not available. GPA: Not available. Number of applicants: 901 instate, 308 out-of-state. Percentage interviewed: 46%. First-year class: 63 men, 11 women; 0% out-of-state. Total enrollment: 143 men, 28 women. Applications: July 1 - October 5 (non-residents), December 1 (residents). Acceptances: July 1 - December 1. Total costs: $4500 instate, $6250 out-of-state.

University of Tennessee Center for the Health Sciences College of Medicine
62 South Dunlap
Memphis, TN 38163

MCAT: VA-550, QA-605, GI-550, Sci-610. GPA: 3.51. Number of applicants: 823 instate. Percentage interviewed: 75%. First-year class: 163 men, 37 women. Total enrollment: 526 men, 84 women. Applications: (Varies) - July 15. Acceptances: January 30 - (varies). Total costs: $4215.

University of Texas Health Science Center at Dallas Southwestern Medical School
5323 Harry Hines Boulevard
Dallas, TX 75235

MCAT: VA-593, QA-629, GI-564, Sci-633. GPA: 3.65. Number of applicants: 1849 instate, 880 out-of-state. Percentage interviewed: 28%. First-year class: 169 men, 33 women; 4.5% out-of-state. Total enrollment: 597 men, 97 women. Applications: June 1 - November 1.

Acceptances: January 15 - September 1. Total costs: $4450 instate, $5050 out-of-state.

University of Texas Health Science Center at San Antonio Medical School
7703 Floyd Curl Drive
San Antonio, TX 78284

MCAT: 583 composite. GPA: 3.5. Number of applicants: 712 instate, 535 out-of-state. Percentage interviewed: 45%. First-year class: 97 men, 31 women; 5% out-of-state. Total enrollment: 398 men, 92 women. Applications: June 1 - November 1. Acceptances: January 15 - until class is enrolled. Total costs: $3870 instate, $4670 out-of-state.

University of Texas Medical Branch at Galveston School of Medicine
Galveston, TX 77550

MCAT: 580 composite. GPA: 3.66. Number of applicants: 1772 instate, 553 out-of-state. Percentage interviewed: 34%. First-year class: 160 men, 46 women; 7% out-of-state. Total enrollment: 614 men, 151 women. Applications: June 1 - November 1. Acceptances: January 15 - until class is enrolled. Total costs: $3305 instate, $4105 out-of-state.

University of Texas Medical School at Houston
Box 20708
Houston, TX 77025

MCAT: QA-629, Sci-599. GPA: 3.4. Number of applicants: 1751 instate, 539 out-of-state. Percentage interviewed: 19%. First-year class: 49 men, 16 women; 7% out-of-state. Total enrollment: 138 men, 30 women. Applications: June 1 - November 1. Acceptances:

January 15 - date of matriculation. Total costs: $2950 instate, $3550 out-of-state.

University of Utah College of Medicine
50 North Medical Drive
Salt Lake City, UT 84132

MCAT: Not available. GPA: Not available. Number of applicants: 329 instate, 1127 out-of-state. Percentage interviewed: 34%. First-year class: 87 men, 14 women; 15% out-of-state. Total enrollment: 352 men, 48 women. Applications: July 1 - November 1. Acceptances: January 15 - March 15. Total costs: $3900 instate, $6050 out-of-state.

University of Vermont College of Medicine
Given Medical Building
Burlington, VT 05401

MCAT: 591 composite. GPA: 3.4. Number of applicants: 103 instate, 2237 out-of-state. Percentage interviewed: 10%. First-year class: 65 men, 19 women; 53% out-of-state (Maine, Massachusetts, & Rhode Island). Total enrollment: 263 men, 64 women. Applications: July 1 - November 1. Acceptances: November 15 - (varies). Total costs: $3900 instate, $6060 out-of-state.

University of Virginia School of Medicine
Box 535
Charlottesville, VA 22901

MCAT: VA-585, QA-635, GI-565, Sci-625. GPA: 3.48. Number of applicants: 704 instate, 2415 out-of-state. Percentage interviewed: 16%. First-year class: 109 men, 29 women; 27% out-of-state. Total enrollment: 425 men, 74 women. Applications: July 1 - November 15.

Acceptances: November 15 - until class is enrolled. Total costs: $3795 instate, $5120 out-of-state.

University of Washington School of Medicine
A-300 Health Sciences Building
Seattle, WA 98195

MCAT: 651 (science). GPA: 3.61. Number of applicants: 432 instate, 1124 out-of-state. Percentage interviewed: 32%. First-year class: 126 men, 49 women; 31% out-of-state. Total enrollment: 442 men, 131 women. Applications: July 1 - December 15. Acceptances: December 15 - September 26. Total costs: $4255 instate, $5585 out-of-state.

University of Wisconsin Medical School
610 North Walnut Street
Madison, WI 53706

MCAT: Not available. GPA: Not available. Number of applicants: 627 instate, 809 out-of-state. Percentage interviewed: 14%. First-year class: 126 men, 33 women; 5% out-of-state. Total enrollment: 487 men, 139 women. Applications: July 1 - December 15. Acceptances: November 15 - (varies). Total costs: $4560 instate, $5710 out-of-state.

Vanderbilt University School of Medicine
Nashville, TN 37232

MCAT: 630 composite. GPA: Not available. Number of applicants: 152 instate, 5222 out-of-state. Percentage interviewed: 28%. First-year class: 64 men, 19 women; 80% out-of-state. Total enrollment: 287 men, 47 women. Applications: July 1 - November 1. Acceptances: December 15 - until class is enrolled. Total costs: $5760.

Washington University School of Medicine
660 South Euclid Avenue
St. Louis, MO 63110

MCAT: VA-593, QA-657, GI-564, Sci-658. GPA: 3.66 (science), 3.60 (nonscience). Number of applicants: 301 instate, 5907 out-of-state. Percentage interviewed: 23%. First-year class: 101 men, 28 women; 83% out-of-state. Total enrollment: 422 men, 119 women. Applications: July 1 - November 1. Acceptances: October 15 - August 25. Total costs: $5900.

Wayne State University School of Medicine
540 East Canfield
Detroit, MI 48201

MCAT: Not available. GPA: Not available. Number of applicants: 1658 instate, 1986 out-of-state. Percentage interviewed: 15%. First-year class: 205 men, 56 women; 2% out-of-state. Total enrollment: 857 men, 167 women. Applications: July 1 - December 15. Acceptances: November 15 - June 30. Total costs: $4600 instate, $6400 out-of-state.

West Virginia University School of Medicine
West Virginia University Medical Center
Morgantown, WV 26506

MCAT: 576 ± 51 composite. GPA: 3.48. Number of applicants: 398 instate, 367 out-of-state. Percentage interviewed: 41%. First-year class: 63 men, 17 women; 0% out-of-state. Total enrollment: 287 men, 50 women. Applications: June 1 - November 30. Acceptances: September 15 - until class is enrolled. Total costs: $2310 instate, $3145 out-of-state.

Wright State University School of Medicine
Dayton, OH 45431

MCAT, GPA, Number of applicants, First-year class, Total enrollment: Not available. Applications: July 1 - November 15. Acceptances: December 15 - until class is enrolled. Total costs: $3650 instate, $5350 out-of-state.

Yale University School of Medicine
333 Cedar Street
New Haven, CT 06510

MCAT: Not available. GPA: Not available. Number of applicants: 200 instate, 1650 out-of-state. Percentage interviewed: 30%. First-year class: 74 men, 28 women; 93% out-of-state. Total enrollment: 314 men, 107 women. Applications: June 1 - November 1. Acceptances: December 15 - March 15. Total costs: $7350.

Notes

Applicants, Applications, and Enrollments

[1]W.F. Dubé. "Woman Students and Woman M.D. Graduates in U.S. Medical Schools for Selected Years from 1914 - 15 to 1972 - 73," *Journal of Medical Education* 48 (1973): 186 - 189.

[2]W.F. Dubé, D.G. Johnson, and B.C. Nelson, "Study of U.S. Medical School Applicants, 1971 - 72," *Journal of Medical Education* 48 (1973): 395-420.

[3]W.F. Dubé, "Applicants for the 1973 - 74 Medical School Entering Class," *Journal of Medical Education* 49 (1974): 1070-1072.

[4]W.F. Dubé, "U.S. Medical School Student Enrollment, 1970 - 71 Through 1974 -75," *Journal of Medical Education* 50 (1975): 303-306.

[5]Ibid., p. 303-306.

[6]T.L. Gordon and W.F. Dubé, "Medical Student Enrollment, 1971 - 72 Through 1975 - 76," *Journal of Medical Education* 51 (1976): 144-146.

The Flexner Report

[1]Abraham Flexner, "Medical Education in the United States and Canada, A Report to the Carnegie Foundation for the Advancement of Teaching," with an introduction by Henry S. Pritchett, in *Bulletin,* 4 (1910), viii.

[2]Ibid., p. x.

[3]Abraham Flexner, "Medical Education 1909 - 1924," in *Education Record* (April, 1924), p. 7.

[4]Ibid., p. 15.

[5]Ibid., p. 11.

[6]Ibid., p. 8.

Bibliography

Tables

"Accredited Medical Schools and Schools of Basic Medical Sciences in the United States, 1974 - 75." *JAMA* 234: 1408-1409.

Dubé, W.F. "Applicants for the 1973 - 74 Medical School Entering Class." *Journal of Medical Education* 49: 1070 - 1072.

―――. "U.S. Medical Student Enrollment, 1970 - 71 Through 1974 - 75." *Journal of Medical Education* 50: 303-306.

―――. "Woman Students and Woman M.D. Graduates in U.S. Medical Schools for Selected Years from 1914 - 15 to 1972 - 73." *Journal of Medical Education* 48: 186-189.

Dubé, W.F., Johnson, D.G., and Nelson, B.C. "Study of U.S. Medical School Applicants, 1971 - 72." *Journal of Medical Education* 48: 395-420.

Gordon, T.L. and Dubé, W.F. "Medical Student Enrollment, 1971 - 72 Through 1975 - 76." *Journal of Medical Education* 51: 144 - 146.

Articles

Flexner, Abraham. "Medical Education in the United States and Canada: A Report to the Carnegie Foundation for the Advancement of Teaching"; introduction by Henry S. Pritchett. *Bulletin* 4: viii.

―――. "Medical Education 1909 - 1924." *Education Record* April, 1924: 7.

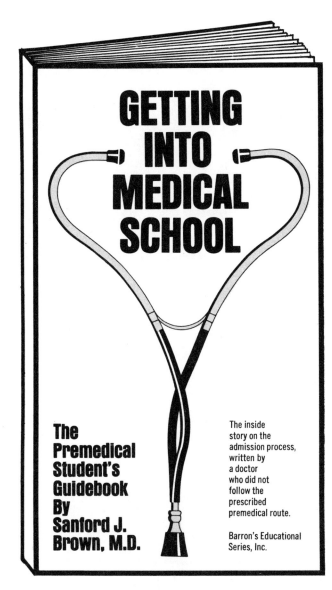

GETTING INTO MEDICAL SCHOOL

The Premedical Student's Guidebook By Sanford J. Brown, M.D.

The inside story on the admission process, written by a doctor who did not follow the prescribed premedical route.

Barron's Educational Series, Inc.

"Majoring in a non-science will probably raise your overall GPA and put you in a more advantageous position when seeking admission . . ."

"Apart from their annual pilgrimage to a medical school (a trip which you can more profitably make on your own), the value of [premedical clubs] is dubious . . ."

"The premedical adviser holds no degree or certification for the job, is not licensed, and is not subject to peer review. The adviser is only as good as personal interest and involvement allow."

The hardest obstacle to overcome in becoming a physician is getting admitted to a medical school. This book cuts through the official jargon and tells you exactly what you really need to do to be accepted. How to choose a college and a major field of study, how to avoid the "Premed Syndrome," how to cope with the MCAT, when, where, and how to apply to medical school, and how to deal with rejections. With a directory of AMA-approved medical schools.

$1.95 paper

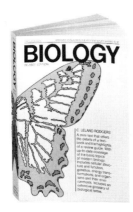
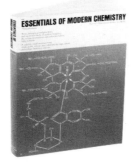
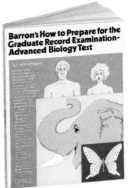
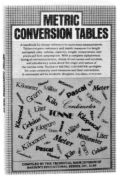
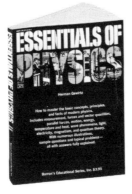
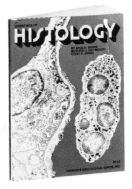